Social Work Practice in Health

Health services practice or working with clients facing health issues requires diverse approaches and wide-ranging knowledge. In this fully revised and expanded second edition, Melissa Petrakis draws on the experience and expertise of leading researchers and practitioners to provide a guide to the disparate settings in which social workers are engaged and the conceptual frameworks and skills needed for effective practice.

Including new chapters on compassion in healthcare, neoliberalism and health, social justice, suicidal distress, and health social work in regional, rural and remote settings, the book begins by examining the nature of health social work and considers its core values and principles. Part I also provides an overview of the social determinants of health. Part II explores key areas of practice including trauma-informed practice, mental health, aged care, dual diagnosis and working with people living with disability. Part III looks at politicised issues, reform agendas in the field including indigenous approaches to health, refugee health, and concludes by considering how a focus on well-being informed by Maori approaches could provide new insights into better practice.

Underpinning the book throughout is a clear guide to assessment procedures, case management, strengths-based practices and developing effective partnerships and collaboration. All this makes *Social Work Practice in Health* a key reference tool for social work students and practitioners.

Melissa Petrakis is an associate professor in social work at Monash University in Melbourne, Australia, and director of SWITCH Research Group. She is a senior research fellow with St Vincent's Hospital Melbourne's Mental Health Service, and has over 30 years' experience in public health and mental health service provision, management and research.

Social Work Practice in Health

An Introduction to Contexts, Theories and Skills

Second Edition

Edited by
Melissa Petrakis

Routledge
Taylor & Francis Group
LONDON AND NEW YORK

Cover image: © Getty Images

Second edition published 2023
by Routledge
4 Park Square, Milton Park, Abingdon, Oxon OX14 4RN

and by Routledge
605 Third Avenue, New York, NY 10158

Routledge is an imprint of the Taylor & Francis Group, an informa business

First edition published by Routledge, 2018

British Library Cataloguing-in-Publication Data
A catalogue record for this book is available from the British Library

Library of Congress Cataloging-in-Publication Data
Names: Petrakis, Melissa, editor.
Title: Social work practice in health : an introduction to contexts, theories and skills / edited by Melissa Petrakis.
Description: 2nd edition. | Abingdon, Oxon ; New York, NY : Routledge, 2023. | Includes bibliographical references and index. |
Identifiers: LCCN 2022025991 (print) | LCCN 2022025992 (ebook) |
ISBN 9781032202709 (hbk) | ISBN 9781032362083 (pbk) | ISBN 9781003330745 (ebk)
Subjects: LCSH: Social service--Australia. | Public health--Australia. | Medical social work--Australia.
Classification: LCC HV473 .S633 2023 (print) | LCC HV473 (ebook) | DDC 361.994--dc23/eng/20220902
LC record available at https://lccn.loc.gov/2022025991
LC ebook record available at https://lccn.loc.gov/2022025992

ISBN: 978-1-032-20270-9 (hbk)
ISBN: 978-1-032-36208-3 (pbk)
ISBN: 978-1-003-33074-5 (ebk)

DOI: 10.4324/9781003330745

Typeset in Sabon
by Taylor & Francis Books

Contents

Illustrations

Figures

Tables

Boxes

Contributors

Carmel Alakus teaches social work at Monash University, having been employed as a social worker for over 40 years. She was a senior social work clinician in adult mental health in an acute inpatient unit, before that at the Academic Unit of North Eastern Metropolitan Psychiatric Service, and in child welfare, health, disability and migrant services.

Amohia Boulton is director of Whakauae Research Services, the only tribally owned health research centre in Aotearoa, and adjunct professor at both Faculty of Health and Environmental Sciences, Auckland University of Technology (AUT) and Health Services Research Centre, Victoria University of Wellington. She is a Māori health researcher from the iwi (tribes) of Ngāti Ranginui, Ngai Te Rangi, Ngāti Pukenga, Ngāti Mutunga and Te Āti Awa o te Waka a Māui.

Lisa Braddy is chief social worker at St Vincent's Hospital Melbourne, Australia, overseeing a team of 30 social workers providing services to acute, sub-acute and palliative care inpatients. She has 25 years' clinical and management experience in health, aged care, disability, community programs and workforce education and training.

Jacinta Chavulak is a senior mental health clinician at The Alfred, and a teaching associate and research assistant at Monash University in Melbourne, Australia. Her direct practice expertise includes emergency psychiatry, suicide prevention, clinical case management, support work and community work.

Melinda Collins is research, quality and data lead within social work at St Vincent's Hospital Melbourne. She has over 20 years' experience as a health social worker, and her primary research interest lies in understanding the lived experience of patients and ensuring their 'voice' and needs of are heard and addressed in all health service responses.

Margaret (Margi) Cowgill is a senior social worker in the mental health service at Peninsula Health, Melbourne. She worked in the United Kingdom in community support teams and hospital-based roles in emergency, orthopaedic/trauma, general medicine, neurology, aged and complex care rehabilitation, and has over 15 years' experience.

Tracey Cropp is a social worker and the kaitakitaki (manager) of the Whānau Support Team at Whanganui Hospice. In her current Whānau Ora practice supervisor position with Hospice, she works with kaimahi to enhance their practice, emotional wellness, and development so that they can in turn effectively support whānau to achieve mauri ora. Tracey is of Te Āti Awa (Taranaki), Ngāti Rūanui (Taranaki), Australian and British descent.

Lynley Cvitanovic is a researcher and evaluator with Whakauae Research, a Ngāti Hauiti owned Māori health research centre based in Whanganui, Aotearoa New Zealand. She is a Pākehā New Zealander of Croatian, English and Irish descent and a social worker and practice supervisor with more than two decades' experience in the community work, mental health, justice, education and public health.

Ros Darracott has 30 years' experience in regional, rural and remote social work in government, non-government, and private practice; in health, mental health, and child and family wellbeing. She has worked in direct service delivery, service design, management and academia and is co-author of *Social Care Practice in Rural Communities* (Federation Press, 2007).

Kate Day is a senior policy advisor with the Victorian Department of Health in Australia, and previously a senior clinical advisor, Office of the Chief Psychiatrist, Victoria's public mental health system. She has over 15 years' direct service provision, project management, policy, service development, team management, mentoring, and staff development expertise.

Niki Edwards is an associate professor of social work at the University of Southern Queensland. She worked in Schools of Medicine at the University of Queensland and Griffith University, and is visiting professor of social work at Fulda University of Applied Sciences in Germany where her teaching, focuses on disability, gender and social inclusion.

Mara Erhardt-Rumpe is general manager service development at the Brotherhood of St Laurence where she oversees service innovation, quality assurance, community engagement, performance and outcomes. She has over 20 years' clinical and management experience in public health, community based services, aged care and disability.

Charlotte Finlayson is a PhD candidate at the University of Sydney, Australia, and works as a social worker in an assertive outreach suicide prevention service in rural and remote New South Wales. She has past experience in the non-government organisations and government sectors providing therapeutic support to people experiencing suicidal distress.

David Hodgson is a senior lecturer in social work at Curtin University. He is associate editor for the journal *Australian Social Work*, and has co-authored (with Lynelle Watts) *Key Concepts and Theory in Social Work* (Palgrave, 2017) and *Social Justice Theory and Practice for Social Work: Critical and Philosophical Perspectives* (Springer, 2019).

Julie King is a senior lecturer and honours coordinator at the Queensland University of Technology in the School of Public Health and Social Work. She is a critical medical anthropologist who has been a social work educator for over ten years, researching across cultures within Australia and the Global South, especially in Southeast Asia and the Pacific.

Rose Knol is a senior social work clinician in the state-wide trauma service, the Victorian Adult Burns service, and the Victorian HIV service, and for 11 years has worked at the Alfred Hospital, Melbourne. She has practised in Melbourne, London and Dublin, and has over 25 years' experience as a social worker in public health, disability and aged care.

Simon Kroes is a senior clinician at Nexus Dual Diagnosis Service at St Vincent's Hospital Melbourne. In 2011 he created the Reasons for Use package (RFUP). In 2016 he won a commendation from Tandem for creating the Carers Can Ask resource. He is chairperson of the North East Dual Diagnosis Youth (NEDDY) Network for best practice in integrated care.

Carrie Lethborg is clinical leader and Senior Social Worker in Health Equity Research at St Vincent's Hospital Melbourne, research fellow in Psycho-oncology at Monash Medical Centre and Senior Lecturer in the Centre for Rural Health, College of Health & Medicine at University of Tasmania. She has over 25 years' experience in oncology.

Debbie Ling is a lecturer in social work at Monash University, research fellow in the Epworth Monash Rehabilitation Medicine Unit and a senior clinician social worker at Epworth HealthCare. She sits on the Australian Compassion Council, Charter for Compassion Australia and the Australia21 Mindful Futures Network Advisory Group.

Penny Lording is a senior social worker at St Vincent's Hospital Melbourne, with responsibility for clinical consultations, education, professional development and supervision. She has extensive experience in mental capacity assessment, safeguarding investigations and community emergency interventions in public hospitals in Melbourne and London, UK.

Kevan Myers is team leader at Nexus Dual Diagnosis Service, St Vincent's Hospital Melbourne where he has been based for over 10 years. He qualified and worked as a social worker in the United Kingdom prior to emigrating to Australia in 1991, and he is a member of the international Motivational Interviewing Network of Trainers (MINT).

Melissa Petrakis is an associate professor in social work at Monash University in Melbourne, Australia, and director of SWITCH Research Group. She is a senior research fellow with St Vincent's Hospital Melbourne's Mental Health Service, and has over 30 years' experience in public health and mental health service provision, management and research.

Kim Robinson is a social work researcher with three decades of national and international expertise working with asylum seekers and refugees. She has published about asylum and refugee mental health, family violence, social justice issues with young unaccompanied minors facing deportation, refugee settlement, and refugee experiences of home and homemaking.

Prue Shanahan is the coordinator of the Koori Beds and coordinates referrals into the Mental Health Acute Inpatient Service, in conjunction with the St Vincent's Aboriginal Health Unit and the Victorian Aboriginal Health Service. She facilitates the provision of culturally safe care in accordance with the Social and Emotional Wellbeing model of care.

Emma Tseris teaches and researches social work in mental health at the University of Sydney. She has practice experience in adult and child and adolescent mental health settings, where she observed diagnostic understandings of distress obscuring social injustices and leading to narrow and often oppressive responses to distress.

Nicole Watt is Aboriginal health care coordinator and team leader of the Aboriginal Hospital Liaison Service at St Vincent's Public Hospital in Melbourne, Australia. She is a proud Yorta Yorta/Wemba Wemba woman, committed to improving Aboriginal and Torres Strait Islander community health outcomes, and a registered nurse with over 20 years' experience.

Lynelle Watts is a senior lecturer in Social Work at Curtin University, Perth, Western Australia. She is the serving president of Australia New Zealand Social Work Welfare Education & Research (ANZSWWER) – a peak body for social work and welfare educators – and is social media editor for the journal *Australian Social Work*.

Preface

Melissa Petrakis

Welcome to this introductory text on health and health services practice. Social work in health is a significant area of social work intervention.

This text provides both a background on health issues and an overview of professional practice knowledge and skills in health and health services. The text describes a number of contemporary approaches to the provision of services to people with health conditions, illnesses, disorders and disabilities. The text examines relevant legislation and ethical issues that influence the provision of these services in the community. Social workers must be alert to such practice issues in order to deliver an effective and appropriate service to the clients, consumers and patients with whom we work.

The structure of the book is a three-part structure. In Part I are four chapters to introduce what health social work is, including role, values and principles for practice. There are then six chapters of health practice and practice contexts in Part II, introducing health work with clients across the lifespan, in acute hospital and community service contexts, and work involving various specialisations. Finally, Part III consists of five chapters highlighting emerging needs in health practice; areas where social work is strongly engaged yet is still working to establish clear approaches and have a meaningful impact due to the changing social and political context.

The aims of the text are to:

- introduce students and new practitioners to health roles, fields, services and settings;
- encourage students and new practitioners to consider specific health problems, to understand and recognise their social and psychological components and consequences, and to consider the broader social and policy dimensions of health problems;
- give attention to those populations who experience vulnerability, the factors used to construct health problems, and the predominating paradigms which influence thinking, understanding, assessment and treatment of health problems;
- explore current knowledge and skills necessary for social work engagement, assessment, intervention and longer-term work with people in a range of health areas; and
- extend understanding of contemporary discourses in settings where health issues predominate.

I encourage student and new practitioner readers to immerse themselves in each chapter of this text, learning about specific populations and work settings, and to also in reading think about key take home messages for practice – in a specific field of health, but also more broadly, in all jobs throughout their social work careers.

Part I

What Is Health Social Work? Role, Values and Principles for Practice

1 An Introduction to Health and Health Services Practice, and the Social Determinants of Health

Melissa Petrakis and Carrie Lethborg

Introduction

Definitions of Health

In 1955 the World Health Organization (WHO) convened a study group to review experience and knowledge on indices and measures for assessment of health, discuss the concept of health and factors affecting health, and basic elements, possible indicators of health, and needs. In their deliberation, published in 1957, importantly they defined health the first key definition of health was provided by the WHO, defining health as 'a condition or quality of the human organism which expressing these adequate functioning of the organism in given conditions, genetic and environmental conditions' (World Health Organization, 1957, p. 8).

This definition represented a significant shift away from a focus on health as a physical or biological condition alone, predominant since the mid-19th century in Western nations (Sheridan & Radmacher, 1992). Health was so defined is no longer solely equated with the absence of illness, and health care with the fight against disease. Health, according to the 1957 WHO definition, was instead defined in terms of *functioning*; so even though individuals may not be in a state of complete physical, or mental, or social wellbeing, if they were functioning adequately then they may be said to be *healthy*. An example of this might be an individual with diabetes who maintains his/her required medications and consequently feels *healthy*, and functions adequately in daily life, and participates in the community.

A medicalised view of health leads to a narrower focus for understanding the complex dimensions which shape health and illness. Grbich (2004) argued that as long as health is seen as entirely biologically determined, and health care conceptualised as the provision of medical services which provide clinical and technological solutions, then important connections between health and the social and economic environments in which it occurs are not made.

Understandings of *health* and *illness* are constantly evolving concepts shaped by prevailing attitudes, beliefs, political, socio-cultural and historical events, social standards and changes to technical and medical knowledge. For example, indigenous health is not a split into the mind/body dichotomy but is holistic and the outcome of a complex interplay between individual, place of birth (and the place of birth of one's ancestors) and spiritual integrity (Grbich 2004). Health practices also vary according to religious practices (e.g. the acceptance or non-acceptance of male and female circumcision). Practices that were acceptable in the 1950s, such as the common practice of removing tonsils without good

DOI: 10.4324/9781003330745-2

cause in children experiencing recurrent throat infections (Hultcrantz & Ericsson 2013), are no longer acceptable today.

Definitions of health and illness, disease and disability are important to enable a common understanding. They are also used in law, in order to decide who is eligible for particular benefits and services (e.g. definitions of disability).

It is important though to consider any definition or diagnostic classification within the context of the assumptions and ideology which underpins it (Frone, Russell & Cooper 1995). So any definition or diagnosis should not be considered in isolation from the social, political, economic or biological circumstances from which it is created, and this includes considerations of the influence of age, gender, culture and ethnicity and individual developmental stage including cognitive, moral, psychosocial and physical factors.

The *Report of the Special Rapporteur on the Right of Everyone to the Enjoyment of the Highest Attainable Standard of Physical and Mental Health* was presented to the Human Rights Council of the United Nations General Assembly in June 2017. In the Introduction, page 3, point 4, it offers a note on terminology:

> 4. Everyone, throughout their lifetime, requires an environment that supports their mental health and wellbeing; in that connection, we are all potential users of mental health services. Many will experience occasional and short-lived psychosocial difficulties or distress that require additional support. Some have cognitive, intellectual and psychosocial disabilities, or are persons with autism who, regardless of self-identification or diagnosis, face barriers in the exercise of their rights on the basis of a real or perceived impairment and are therefore disproportionately exposed to human rights violations in mental health settings. Many may have a diagnosis related to mental health or identify with the term, while others may choose to identify themselves in other ways, including as survivors.
>
> (United Nations General Assembly Human Rights Council, 2017, p. 3)

Prevailing Assumptions about Health and Illness

It is important to consider:

- What assumptions does this society makes about health and illness?
- Who has been influential in developing these assumptions or standards and how have they become commonly accepted?

Some prevailing assumptions include:

- *People choose to be sick or well.* This belief is located in deviancy models (Kleinman, 1978), whereby people are said to be motivated to be sick in order to be able to be dependent. The belief here is that disease arises because there is something intrinsically wrong with the individual, as the body is an extension and expression of the inner self. Aspects of this belief system are seen in positions taken for example on chronic fatigue syndrome, where some health professionals believed it was a psychosomatic condition (Ware, 1992) because they could find no physical evidence of its existence using standard medical testing.
- *It is best to express dis-ease through physical conditions.* This illustrates the mind-body split where physical disease is treated as more acceptable than emotional

disease. Society can confer a degree of acceptability on illness – the sick role – which may encourage people to express life problems physiologically and seek medical solutions for them; e.g. 'Mediterranean back' (Rubinstein, 1982) or Munchausen by proxy. Some alternative health groups have utilised this belief positively, focusing on the benefits of relaxation, mediation and diet as ways of healing the inner self and therefore the expressed illness.

Each society determines what it regards as normal or healthy and these decisions change over time. For example, childbirth in the 1940s through to the1960s took on the characteristics of illness as hospitals and medical services took over responsibility for childbirth. This could be said to be a response to high levels of mortality and the availability of services to safely deliver children. But it could also be understood in terms of the dominance and emergence of particular professions, such as obstetricians over midwives, and the cultural dominance of taking childbirth out of the realm of women and the family. Associated with this there was also an increased use of pain relief and caesarean. Attitudes to childbirth today are significantly different, and pregnancy and childbirth are seen as health states not illness. This change may have been influenced by healthier women, the feminist movement, consumer rights movement, escalating hospital costs and the emergence of economic rationalism.

Patterns of Health and Illness

The social organisation of society is closely connected with health and illness, and we know from mortality and morbidity studies that different patterns of social organisation produce different health and illness profiles. So an individual's health status is not just a result of physical health, or the presence or absence of disease, it is the consequence of the interaction between lifestyle, biological, environmental and socio-cultural factors.

The Ottawa Charter for Health Promotion addressed health in terms of social capital:

> To reach a state of complete physical mental and social wellbeing, an individual or group must be able to identify and to realize aspirations, to satisfy needs, and to change or cope with the environment. Health is, therefore, seen as a resource for everyday life, not the objective of living. Health is a positive concept emphasizing social and personal resources, as well as physical capacities. Therefore, health promotion is not just the responsibility of the health sector, but goes beyond healthy lifestyles to wellbeing.
>
> The fundamental conditions and resources for health are peace, shelter, education, food, income, a stable ecosystem, sustainable resources, social justice and equity.
>
> Improvement in health requires a secure foundation in these basic prerequisites.
>
> The enjoyment of the highest attainable standard of health is one of the fundamental rights of every human being without distinction of race, religion, political belief, economic or social condition.
>
> (World Health Organization, 1986, article 57)

This Charter clearly outlines what is required to achieve good health, if adequate resources exist.

In Australia there is relatively good health status, with the exception of groups with more disadvantages such as the indigenous population (discussed in Chapter 12), refugees in detention (discussed in Chapter 14) and some older people (discussed in Chapter 8). Improvements in public health measures, socioeconomic conditions and education, particularly through health promotion campaigns, have produced an overall increased lifespan in our society (Australian Institute of Health and Welfare, 2017). Public health initiatives have eradicated many epidemic diseases and now many diseases of concern are those related to lifestyle changes over the most recent two generations; for example: respiratory illness, heart disease, accidents and obesity (Zammit, Liddicoat, Moonsie & Makker, 2010). Public health promotion campaigns that have been influential on our thinking about health and illness in Australia have included: the *Quit* campaign; the *Safe Sex* campaigns, including the *Grim Reaper* AIDS campaign of the 1980s; Beyondblue, the national depression initiative; and the *Slip slop slap* campaign, concerned with skin cancer prevention.

Many chronic illnesses are also illnesses of ageing, and with increased lifespan yet falling fertility rates there is a proportional increase in the aged in our societies in Western industrialised nations. In Australia 35% of the population (7 million people) suffers from one or more chronic illnesses; asthma, type 2 diabetes, coronary heart disease, cerebrovascular disease (largely stroke), arthritis, osteoporosis, COPD, depression or high blood pressure for example, arthritis, hypertension, asthma, and migraine (Australian Institute of Health and Welfare, 2014). These are large numbers of people and are conditions largely managed in the community; social work potentially has an important role here.

Epidemiology offers much of this information about patterns of illness. It deals with the incidence, aetiology (cause), distribution, effects and control of disease in populations. It has been pivotal in providing information about the relationship between risk factors such as smoking and lung cancer, drinking infected water and disease, and unsafe sexual practices and sexually transmitted diseases. More recently it has extended its boundaries from the purely physical diseases to social contributors to disease and illness such as the effect of gender, poverty, culture and class.

A Focus on the Social Determinants of Health

More recently a conceptual shift has enabled us to understand the importance of the *social determinants* of health, 'the conditions in which people are born, grow, live, work and age and including the health system' (World Health Organization, 2005). This perspective notes the sensitivity of health to the social environment, and brings a new complexity to our understanding of health and wellbeing – especially in relation to discrepancies amongst populations (Marmot, 2005). 'It is not simply that poor material circumstances are harmful to health', Wilkinson and Marmot state, 'the social meaning of being poor, unemployed, socially excluded or otherwise stigmatised also matters' (Wilkinson & Marmot, 2003, p. 9).

Social determinants explain inequalities of health *within* and *between* communities and countries. A 20-year life expectancy gap between Indigenous and non-Indigenous people in Australia for example (Australian Bureau of Statistics, 2013a), cannot be explained simply in relation to economics without an understanding of the influence of a wide range of factors (Calma, 2005). The WHO includes the following list in its description of the social determinants of health (Wilkinson & Marmot, 2003):

- the social gradient;
- stress;
- early life;
- social exclusion;

- work;
- unemployment;
- social support;
- addiction;
- food; and
- transport.

These factors present a multifaceted web of social and environmental influences that assist in explaining health discrepancies and directing policy makers in their response to such discrepancies.

According to social work academic Professor Paul Bywaters, tackling health inequalities is a major new challenge for social work, putting forward four main points for his case (Bywaters, 2007) that:

1 Health inequalities are a matter of social justice and human rights.
2 The causes of health inequalities are primarily social.
3 Poverty and poor health are common characteristics of social work service users.
4 Therefore health inequalities are a vital issue for social workers in all settings.

Indeed, social work is proud of its micro and macro focus on issues as a point of difference among health care professions as it enables an understanding of the inexplicable links between social determinants and health and the possible reasons for the inequality of outcomes and access to care.

The WHO's Commission on Social Determinants of Health (CSDH) (World Health Organization, 2005) suggested three overarching recommendations in response to the inequities of health outcomes:

1 Improve daily living conditions.
2 Tackle the inequitable distribution of power, money, and resources.
3 Measure and understand the problem and assess the impact of action.

Later reviews and commissions, or calls for commissions, have suggested these remain key concerns (Marmot, Allen, Bell, Bloomer & Goldblatt, 2012). These recommendations illustrate the complexity of both the *causes* of health inequalities and the *responses* required to address them. Understanding the breadth of inequality and its impact on health is an important first step for any social worker, in particular the experience of social exclusion and the avoidable nature of the different opportunities available to members of our society.

The United Nations Special Rapporteur report mentioned earlier acknowledges the context globally as:

> Despite clear evidence that there can be no health without mental health, nowhere in the world does mental health enjoy parity with physical health in national policies and budgets or in medical education and practice. Globally, it is estimated that less than 7 per cent of health budgets is allocated to address mental health. In lower-income countries, less than $2 per person is spent annually on it (PLOS Medicine Editors 2013; World Health Organization, 2014). Most investment is focused on long-term institutional care and psychiatric hospitals, resulting in a near total policy

> failure to promote mental health holistically for all (World Health Organization, 2014). The arbitrary division of physical and mental health and the subsequent isolation and abandonment of mental health has contributed to an untenable situation of unmet needs and human rights violations (see A/HRC/34/32, paras. 11–21), including of the right to the highest attainable standard of mental and physical health (World Health Organization, 2016).
>
> (United Nations General Assembly Human Rights Council, 2017, p. 3, point 6)

Social Exclusion

Central to the role of social determinants in relation to health is the exclusion of those living in disadvantaged situations from the wider society. In particular, this aspect of disadvantage impacts directly on access to services but also has broader implications. Having access to fewer economic resources directly impacts on the amount of social participation that can be enjoyed and leads to 'social exclusion'. Social exclusion is 'the failure of society to provide certain individuals and groups with those rights and benefits normally available to its members, such as employment, adequate housing, health care, education and training, etc'. Kawachi and Berkman (2001) show the breadth of the impact of 'social exclusion' to include restrictions around consumption, production, political engagement as well as social interaction (see Table 1.1).

The impact of social exclusion then, encompasses a person's access to work, support services, connection to family, friends and community as well as their ability to manage personal crises and to have their needs and concerns recognised (Australian Social Inclusion Board, 2010).

While social exclusion and economic inequities are linked they cannot be totally explained by each other. Indeed, decisions about *what* resources are needed to relieve material deprivation as well as *who* gets these resources are socially determined (Kim et al., 2000). Thus, while considered a Right according to the Universal Declaration of Human Rights (United Nations, 1984), being able to participate in society, connect to and support others, maintain a role, claim a status, access support and feel a sense of belonging, is in fact not available to all. This denial to simply be a part of the way of life experienced by others has a broad impact and can be socially and psychologically damaging, costly as well as being harmful to health (Kawachi et al., 1997).

Thus health and wellbeing is influenced not only by the individual genetic makeup of aa person but the social factors they are subject to. These social factors influence not only physical health but also access to a wider social world, to a sense of belonging and to an overall sense of wellbeing.

Table 1.1 Ways that social exclusion impacts on individuals' lives

Consumption	*The incapacity to purchase goods and services relative to need*
Production	A lack of participation in economically or socially valued activities
Political engagement	A lack of participation within government processes (local, state, federal decision making)
Social interaction	A lack of connectedness to family, friends and the community in which one lives

Source: Australian Social Inclusion Board (2010)

Intersectionality

As social work in the health setting faces an increasingly complex world of chronic illness, social determinants of health and trauma informed frameworks, the need to understand the 'person in environment' is more important than ever. The cultural, ethnic, biological, political and economic factors that make up many of the groups of people we work with are increasingly overlapping, resulting in experiences of multiple inequities (Bernard, 2020). A person with intersecting diversities could be discriminated against, consciously or unconsciously because of racism, sexism, ageism, classism, ableism and so on.

Intersectionality refers to the way that multiple forms of oppression can be experienced when minority identities overlap (Cole, 2009) and offers a framework to consider power, oppression and justice at multiples levels. Simon, Boyd and Subica (2022) consider that social work education should 'shift from educating students to evaluate diverse clients as the accumulation of individual identities operating in isolation (e.g., race or ethnicity, gender, sexual orientation) to recognizing how these identities intersect to influence health and wellbeing based on these identities' shared roots in oppression and privilege'.

Indeed, given that these identifying factors influence how people are viewed and the power or powerlessness they experience as a result, social workers also need to reflect on their own biases and world views and how this influences their work. Sylvia Duckworth's wheel of power/privilege (Figure 1.1) offers an effective model for identifying where one 'fits' in relation to privilege, power and vulnerability. The closer a person's characteristics

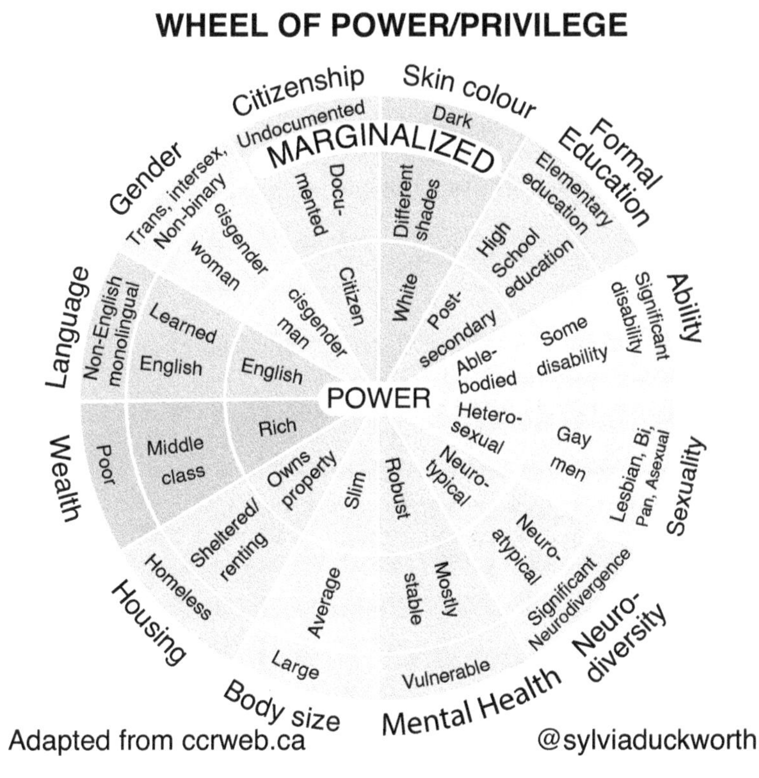

Figure 1.1 Sylvia Duckworth's wheel of power/privilege

are to the centre of the wheel, the more power they may experience in their lives. This is also an important way to understand how these different factors can interact and intersect to influence our own practice as social workers.

The Role of Social Work

Social workers need to understand health and wellbeing, ill health, disability and disease because:

- The health and social problems of the individuals and families with whom we work are often inextricably interrelated.
- Individuals/families/groups/communities often present with problems which involve health issues.
- Social workers are both consumers and carers and to work effectively with clients and other professionals, we must be informed about health.
- By participating in health care, social workers can contribute professionally to the prevailing debates, drawing on their social work ethics and values.

The Skills Social Workers Bring to the Area of Health

Social workers bring a number of skills to the area of health care provision. They include:

- Systemic thinking.
- Politics – internal and external (own and those of your organisation and government).
- Professional ethics, including:
    - respect for human dignity and worth;
    - pursuit of social justice;
    - demonstrated through service to humanity;
    - integrity; and
    - competence.
- Direct Practice skills:
    - assessment, planning, intervention, goal attainment, evaluation and termination plus the associated micro skills;
    - a critical mind and ability to be self-critical;
    - knowledge of human development;
    - knowledge of sociology and social theory;
    - skills in working with groups and networks;
    - understanding of policy, planning and programming; and
    - passion and idealism.

Challenges to Social Workers

The role of the health service practitioner has changed over the last few decades and there is more emphasis for social workers to be multi-skilled. This has been influenced by case mix and the reduction in differentiation of skills (Patford, 1999).

These changes put pressure on the social work profession to:

- project our identity through demonstrating competence and demarcating our occupational turf;
- increase our research base in the qualitative area and the evidence base of reports on successful social work interventions; and
- demonstrate interventions improve outcomes at a reasonable cost.

Social work will increasingly have a greater role in ambulatory care (i.e. non-hospital-based care, shorter hospital stays, self-management programs, peer training and aged care).

There will be increasing focus on the most vulnerable groups rather than those in need of support. This has and will continue to involve a gradual shift from hospital based social work to community based social work. There will be an increase in private practice which has not traditionally been the domain of social workers. Associated with this will be the accreditation of social workers so they may receive Medicare payments.

Dominelli et al. (2001, pp. 1–2) caution:

> Understanding the nature of the changes that are reframing social work locally, nationally and internationally is crucial if social work is to survive as a discipline and practice making a worthwhile contribution to human wellbeing. Responding to this becomes a challenge that requires social work educators and practitioners to rethink their approach to social work to develop theories and forms of practice that can use the profession's existing strengths particularly its capacity for critical, reflexive practice, to move in directions that are consistent with a value base rooted to promoting human rights and social justice in and through practice.

Social Disadvantage

Within Australia these factors explain some of the unacceptable discrepancies in health outcomes for Aboriginal and Torres Strait Islanders. Indeed, we cannot consider the needs of an Aboriginal person without considering the context of social disadvantage. Aboriginal and Torres Strait Islander people have been reported to be the most disadvantaged of all Australians (Australian Government, 1998). As a group, they are disadvantaged relative to other Australians with respect to a number of socioeconomic factors, and these disadvantages place them at greater risk of ill health and reduced wellbeing.

Indeed, two thirds (77%) of Aboriginal people (Australian Bureau of Statistics, 2006), as compared to 59% of the total population report that they experienced one or more significant stressors in the previous 12 months and this population are twice as likely as their non-Aboriginal counterparts to feel high or very high levels of psychological distress (Australian Bureau of Statistics, 2006).

Conclusion

When working with people from vulnerable situations in health care – those who are homeless, living with drug addiction and/or mental health issues, are migrant and/or do not speak English and Aboriginal and Torres Strait islanders – the social worker must bring the understanding of context from a social, historical and political viewpoint in order to fully comprehend individual experiences. Advocacy must be included in both clinical and academic work so that social work is providing a voice for the voiceless and drawing the threads of inequality and health outcomes together, to prevent the vulnerable being blamed and solutions being narrow. As Professor Bywaters (2007, p. 366) states, 'addressing health inequalities implies that social work has to become more actively engaged with critical global social, economic, environmental and political issues'.

Key Website Resources

Australian Institute of Health and Welfare (www.aihw.gov.au) The nation's premier source of statistics and informed commentary on: patterns and determinants of health and illness; health across the life stages; the provisions and use of health services; health expenditure and workforce; and health sector performance.

National Health Priority Areas of the Australian Government www.aihw.gov.au/nhpa/index.cfm

National Health Priority Areas of the New Zealand Government (www.health.govt.nz/new-zealand-health-system/health-targets).

World Health Organization (www.who.int/en).

References

Australian Bureau of Statistics (2006) *National Aboriginal and Torres Strait Islander Health Survey: Australia, 2004–2005*. Canberra: Australian Bureau of Statistics.

Australian Bureau of Statistics (2013a). *Life Tables for Aboriginal and Torres Strait Islander Australians, 2010–2012*. Cat. no. 3302.0.55.003. Canberra: Australian Bureau of Statistics.

Australian Bureau of Statistics (2013b). *Australian Aboriginal and Torres Strait Islander Health Survey: First Results, Australia, 2012–2013*. Cat. no. 4727.0.55.001. Canberra: Australian Bureau of Statistics.

Australian Government (1998). *Australian Report to the Human Rights Commission*. CCPR/C/AUS/98/3. Human Rights Commission.

Australian Institute of Health and Welfare (2014). *Australia's Health 2014*. Canberra: Australian Institute of Health and Welfare.

Australian Institute of Health and Welfare (2017). *Ageing*. Canberra: Australian Institute of Health and Welfare. Retrieved from www.aihw.gov.au/ageing.

Australian Social Inclusion Board (2010). *Annual Report*. Australian Social Inclusion Board.

Bernard, C (2020). Why intersectionality matters for social work practice in adult services, ageing, knowledge and skills, society, social work with adults. Retrieved from https://socialworkwithadults.blog.gov.uk/2020/01/31/why-intersectionality-matters-for-social-work-practice-in-adult-services/

Bywaters P (2007). Tackling inequalities in health: a global challenge for social work. *British Journal of Social Work*, 39(2), 353–367.

Calma T (2005). *Aboriginal and Torres Strait Islander Social Justice Commission*. Sydney: Human Rights and Equal Opportunity Commission.

Cole, E R (2009). Intersectionality and research in psychology. *American Psychologist*, 64(3), 170–180.

Dominelli L, Lorenz W & Soydan H (2001). *Beyond Racial Divides: Ethnicities in Social Work practice*. Farnham: Ashgate.

Frone M R, Russell M & Cooper M L (1995). Relationship of work and family stressors to psychological distress: the independent moderating influence of social support, mastery, active coping, and self-focused attention. In R Crandall & P L Perrewe (eds), *Occupational Stress: A Handbook*, 129–150. Boca Raton, FL: CRC Press.

Grbich, C. (2004). *Health in Australia: Sociological Concepts and Issues* (3rd edition). Pearson Australia.

Hultcrantz E & Ericsson E (2013). Factors influencing the indication for tonsillectomy: a historical overview and current concepts. *ORL*, 75(3), 184–191.

Kawachi I & Berkman L F. (2001). Social ties and mental health. *Journal of Urban Health: Bulletin of the New York Academy of Medicine*, 78(3), 458–467.

Kawachi I, Kennedy B, Lochner K, Prothrow-Stith D (1997). Social capital, income inequality and mortality. *American Journal of Public Health*; 87(9), 1491–1498.

Kim J, Mullen J, Irwin A & Gershman J (2000). *Dying for Growth: Global Inequality and the Health of the Poor*. Monroe, ME: Common Courage Press.

Kleinman A (1978). Concepts and a model for the comparison of medical systems as cultural systems. *Social Science & Medicine, Part B: Medical Anthropology*, 12, 85–93.

Koenig H (1995). Use of acute services and mortality among religious and non-religious copers with medical illness. *Journal of Religious Gerentology*, 9, 1–22.

Marmot M (2005). Social determinants of health inequalities. *Lancet*, 365(9464), 1099–1104.

Marmot M, Allen J, Bell R, Bloomer E & Goldblatt P (2012). WHO European review of social determinants of health and the health divide. *Lancet*, 380(9846), 1011–1029.

Patford J (1999). What's happening in health: progress and prospects for social work. *Australian Social Work*, 52(1), 3–7.

PLOS Medicine Editors (2013). The paradox of mental health: over-treatment and under-recognition, *PLOS Medicine*, 10(5).

Rubinstein A (1982). Mediterranean back and other stereotypes: a review of the Australian literature dealing with industrial back injuries. *The Australian Journal of Social Issues*, 17(4), 295.

Sheridan C L & Radmacher S A (1992). *Health Psychology: Challenging the Biomedical Model*. John Wiley & Sons.

Simon J D, Boyd R, Subica A M (2022). Refocusing intersectionality in social work education: creating a brave space to discuss oppression and privilege. *Journal of Social Work Education*, 58(1), 34–45.

Thomas K (2003). *Religion and the Decline of Magic: Studies in Popular Beliefs in Sixteenth and Seventeenth-Century England*. London: Penguin.

United Nations (1984). The universal declaration of human rights. Retrieved from www.un.org/en/documents/udhr/.

United Nations General Assembly Human Rights Council (2017). *Report of the Special Rapporteur on the Right of Everyone to the Enjoyment of the Highest Attainable Standard of Physical and Mental Health*. A/HRC/35/21. Retrieved from https://ap.ohchr.org/documents/dpage_e.aspx?si=A/HRC/35/21.

Ware N C (1992). Suffering and the social construction of illness: the delegitimation of illness experience in chronic fatigue syndrome. *Medical Anthropology Quarterly*, 6(4), 347–361.

Wilkinson R G & Marmot M (2003). *Social Determinants of Health: The Solid Facts*. Second edition. Geneva: World Health Organization.

World Health Organization (1957). *Measurement of Levels of Health: Report of a Study Group*. Technical Report Series, 137. Geneva: World Health Organization.

World Health Organization (1986). *The Ottawa Charter for Health Promotion*. Geneva: World Health Organization.

World Health Organization (2005). *Commission on Social Determinants of Health, World Health Organization*. Geneva: World Health Organization. Retrieved from www.who.int/social_determinants/thecommission/en/.

World Health Organization (2014). *Mental Health Atlas*. Geneva: World Health Organization.

World Health Organization (2016). Living in hell: abuses against people with psychosocial disabilities in Indonesia. *Human Rights Watch*, March.

Zammit C, Liddicoat H, Moonsie I & Makker H (2010). Obesity and respiratory diseases. *International Journal of General Medicine*, 3(3), 335–343.

2 A Social Justice Perspective on the Bio-Psycho-Social-Spiritual Dimensions of Health

Lynelle Watts and David Hodgson

Introduction

This chapter explores a social justice perspective on the bio-psycho-social-spiritual dimensions of health and wellbeing. Social justice is a core value and guiding principle of social work, and striving for social justice is important to human health. Social justice involves questions over the socio-political organisation of society, including how and on what basis social resources are distributed, human rights, and people's access to decision-making processes that impact on their health and their wellbeing (Watts & Hodgson, 2019). Social justice can give a meta-ethical purpose to social workers practising in health contexts, particularly to make improvements in the social determinants of health that shape different health outcomes across the population. This chapter discusses social justice in light of a holistic view of human health, by applying in a bio-psycho-social-spiritual conceptual framework. It explains the theoretical principles and practice implications that underpin social work thinking in relation to human health, understood as a biological, psychological, social and spiritual phenomena.

Social justice and health

As reflected in social work ethical codes internationally, social justice is a core value and guiding principle of social work (Australian Association of Social Workers, 2020; National Association of Social Workers, 2015; British Association of Social Workers, 2012). Social justice concerns the socio-political organisation of society, including how and on what basis social resources are distributed, human rights, and people's access to decision-making processes that impact on their health and their wellbeing (Watts & Hodgson, 2019). The Australian Association of Social Workers Code of Ethics, defines the pursuit of social justice as follows:

> The social work profession: promotes justice and social fairness, by acting to reduce barriers and to expand choice and potential for all persons, with special regard for those who are disadvantaged, vulnerable, oppressed or have exceptional needs … advocates change to social systems and structures that preserve inequalities and injustice … opposes and works to eliminate all violations of human rights and affirms that civil and political rights must be accompanied by economic, social and cultural rights … promotes the protection of the natural environment as inherent to social wellbeing … promotes community participation in societal processes and decisions and in the development and implementation of social policies and services.
> (Australian Association of Social Workers, 2020, p. 9)

DOI: 10.4324/9781003330745-3

The AASW definition of social justice points to a moral consideration for the most disadvantaged, and a perspective that takes into account people's experiences and circumstances within a wider social, political, economic and cultural context. When thinking about human health, our orientation is necessarily at the intersections between individual health, and the contexts of people's experiences and needs. For example, it is well established that early mortality, morbidity, disability and ill-health disproportionately affect people who are poor and socially and/or economically disadvantaged (Marmot, 2005).

Hence, the attainment of social justice is commensurate with meeting human health needs. The Ottawa Charter for Health Promotion (World Health Organization, 1986) lists social justice and equity as among several fundamental conditions necessary for human health. A good proportion of the Sustainable Development Goals (SDGs) directly relate to social justice (e.g. poverty reduction, addressing gender inequities, inequality reduction, improving access to justice, health, and liveable communities). The interrelation between social justice, human rights and health is increasingly being recognised as fundamental to public health programs and strategies (McKay & Taket, 2020), because as Marmot et al. (2008) argue, 'social injustice is killing people on a grand scale, and the reduction of health inequities, between and within countries, is an ethical imperative' (p. 1661).

Many health problems emergent during the time of industrialisation and urbanisation were arguably the product of the environment (e.g. poor housing, overcrowding, dirty water, lack of sewerage, and the health problems caused by dirty industry). Social reformist movements called upon governments to invest in infrastructure and public health initiatives to improve the conditions of living. Venkatapuram (2011, p. 4) contends that human beings experience health and illness as an outcome from an interaction between 'internal biological endowments and needs that change over the lifecourse, individual behaviours and external physical environment and social conditions'. The fact that social conditions might play a confounding role in preventing a person from flourishing – and indeed causing suffering (of many kinds) – is a prospect we should find especially disturbing. Social conditions are those aspects of human life that should be in the purview of social institutions and, as such, these social institutions are part of the machinery of government. Accordingly, social workers are called upon to 'recognise the impact of the environment on the physical and mental health and wellbeing of people and its fundamental importance to the future of human society' (Australian Association of Social Workers, 2020, p. 13).

A social justice orientation can give a meta-ethical purpose to social workers practising in health contexts, particularly to make improvements to the social determinants of health that shape different health outcomes across the population. There is a moral purpose to this: human beings are beings that have concerns and cares, and therefore, we are capable of flourishing *and* suffering (Sayer, 2011). Human beings are also able to understand the various conditions that cause suffering as well as those that might enable flourishing: we are capable of being reflexive about these conditions (Archer, 2007). Venkatapuram (2011, p. 1) observes that 'for human beings to be able to live a full lifespan and experience as few avoidable physical and mental impairments as possible they need to be surrounded by a supportive environment'.

The basic features of such an environment go beyond access to medical care – they direct our attention to the broad range of conditions that can impact on health. These are access to shelter, nutritious food, clean water, emotional nurturing and care, environments that include physical and cognitive stimulation and protection from different forms of violence and abuse (Venkatapuram, 2011). Economist and philosopher Amartya Sen

(2002, p. 659) puts health and illness at the centre of any discussion of justice because we 'must come to grips with the larger issue of fairness and justice in social arrangements, including economic allocations, paying appropriate attention to the role of health in human life and freedom.'

This calls on social work to embed principles of social justice, somewhat regardless of field or practice setting, as an ethical duty as a support for people's health. We can consider what this might look like by using a social justice framework developed by Watts and Hodgson (2019). The framework has four components that can be considered as crucial elements for social justice-informed social work practice: a critical perspective; a distributive perspective; issues of rights and autonomy; and, participation and decision-making (Watts & Hodgson, 2019).

- A critical perspective means that social workers must pay attention to, and contest, relations of domination and oppression that create misrecognition, violence, powerlessness, forms of cultural imperialism, marginalisation and exploitation (Young, 1990).
- A distributive perspective means that social workers need to work for publicly accountable institutions for the fair and equal distribution of society's goods and resources whether material, symbolic, or economic.
- A rights and autonomy perspective relates to supporting 'people to act as moral agents with dignity, worth, and in recognition of their rights as human beings with personal and social identities' (Watts & Hodgson, 2019, p. 173).
- Participation and decision making calls on social workers to 'increase the spaces for participation and democratic decision-making, discussion, debate and inclusion in public discourse' (Watts & Hodgson, 2019, p 173).

The following section explains the key theoretical underpinnings of a bio-psycho-social-spiritual perspective in health as it relates to social justice.

Towards a Bio-Psycho-Social-Spiritual Perspective on Health

Social work is defined by its person-in-environment perspective, and a key technique of practice, which broadly accords with this perspective, is a psycho-social assessment (sometimes called a biopsychosocial assessment). A psycho-social assessment is a collaborative process used to gather information, organise that information coherently, make informed judgements and assessments, and plan and justify courses of action. According to the Australian Association of Social Workers *Psychosocial Assessments Scope of Practice* (2015), a psychosocial assessment explores the 'physical, psychological and social aspects of the client and their situation. This includes problems and strengths in social role functioning; in meeting financial and other basic needs; in family interactions, significant relationships and other social supports, and cultural factors' (Australian Association of Social Workers, 2015, p. 3). In an extension of this model, some argue that spiritual aspects should be included, in what has been termed a bio-psycho-social-spiritual assessment (Hunt, 2014).

Human beings have very particular evolved *needs* that require fulfilment if we are to achieve flourishing and avoid unnecessary suffering. We have biological needs, psychological needs, social needs, and to some extent, spiritual needs. Broadly, these needs include: adequate nutritional food and clean water; adequate protective housing; a non-hazardous work environment; a non-hazardous physical environment; appropriate health care; security in childhood; significant primary relationships (e.g. supportive groups, close and confiding relationships); physical security; economic security; education; and, safe birth control and child bearing (Doyal & Gough, 1991).

Although these needs are picked up in a bio-psycho-social-spiritual framework, they are concomitant with a social justice ethic and person-in-environment perspective in social work.

What Does the *Bio* in a Bio-Psycho-Social-Spiritual Assessment Refer to?

When assessing for human biological needs, we may focus on things like physical health, diet, sleep, alcohol and other drugs, and medications. These are important considerations, but are narrowly concerned with individual functioning; on their own they do not obviously connect to the social context of human biological needs. Corning (2005), writing in the field of systems theory, bio-economics and evolutionary biology, contends that the primary adaptive and evolutionary functions of what people need in the physiological sense are foundational to individual and species survival and adaptation. He calls this the survival indicators framework, and has identified a scope of biological characteristics that are 'irreducible functional requisites for biological adaptation in the human species' (p. 283). These elements are non-arbitrary and interrelated: the basic biological needs of individuals are at the same time indicators of population well-being. In other words, individual biological needs are determined by, and representative of, the biological (and social justice) conditions of whole populations. They are as follows:

- **Thermoregulation** – the ability to maintain consistent body temperature. Culturally, people have found ways to do this adaptively, such as building shelter, clothes, and things like air conditioning systems.
- **Waste elimination** – what Corning is talking about is eliminating waste produced by groups of people – household and industrial waste for example, and the systems that are needed to safely remove and dispose of them.
- **Nutrition** – an appropriate spectrum of a balanced diet of macros and an acceptable mix of vitamins and minerals, and the agricultural and distributive systems that feed people (food security).
- **Water** – access to uncontaminated water for drinking, but also for hygiene, food processing and preparation, waste disposal, etc. Clean water is elementary to other basic needs, and hence when it is compromised it has a negative flow on effect to other needs.
- **Mobility** – the ability to change location geographically. It is a primary need important to satisfy other needs, and mobility allows people to adapt to changing personal, geographical, economic, political circumstances. The restriction of human mobility threatens this adaptive need.
- **Sleep** – adequate quality sleep is necessary for physical and mental health; however, various aspects of human societies may interfere with it (e.g. work, stress, late television, insomnia, noisy environments).
- **Respiration** – clean oxygenated air. Some household and work environments, air pollution and modern habitations may affect this basic need.
- **Physical safety** – which means avoiding physical injury or death. This is greatly affected by personal and also circumstantial and environmental factors. The social and cultural responses here are very complex involving elaborate approaches to mitigate the potential and actual causes of injury and death.

- **Physical health** – includes the absence of metabolic or genetic problems as well as the absence of physically debilitating conditions, which may be environmental (such as diseases) and personal (such as lifestyle behaviours).
- **Mental health** – this is defined as a 'state of mind that allows an individual to carry on normal functioning and self-care without significant impairment (harm)' (Corning, 2005, p. 293). What Corning is saying is that as a basic need, mental health should be such that it allows someone to live in a way that does not impact 'life sustaining activity' (ibid., p. 293).
- **Communications** – 'the ability to transmit and receive information from the environment … [which] is a fundamental property of all complex organisms' (ibid., p. 294). In human societies, communications are indelibly complex and include a vast range of kinds of information as well as different methods for distributing and receiving it. The litmus test for information and communication is the extent to which it helps or hinders normal functioning and meeting instrumental adaptive needs.
- **Social relationships** – social relationships are key to accessing information, which is important to normal functioning and survival. Social relationships can be protective and nurturing but they must – if they are to be functional – contain social values that are not harmful (e.g. not abusive, exploitative, alienating).
- **Reproduction** – there are two aspects relevant to social work that need to be considered here if reproduction is to be sustained as a functional basic need: (1) maternal health from conception to the health of the mother and foetus to birth itself (which may necessitate access to health services, nutrition, medical assessments and prenatal and postnatal care); and, (2) resourcing and managing the conflict that invariably arises between parental needs and child needs (i.e. parenting support over potentially competing interests and priorities).
- **Nurturance of offspring** – Corning attests this is the 'culmination of the process of adaptation' (ibid., p. 297) because it requires all the other needs to be optimally present if this is to be effectively satisfied. Young children require all these other needs, but they also require very specific developmental needs (e.g. cognitive, educational, emotional, and attachment).

These biological needs are universal, but the methods and means of meeting these needs vary according to cultural, social, geographical and historical factors. For example, nurturance of offspring is a human basic need, but *how* this happens may be subject to considerable variation and cultural disagreement. Applying these biological needs to the context of bio-psycho-social-spiritual assessments can help us broach questions of social justice, because although these are individual needs, they are at the same time a reflection of population health and the (in)adequacy of social and economic systems to support them.

What Does the *Psycho* in a Bio-Psycho-Social-Spiritual Assessment Refer to?

Psychology is not one thing but instead encompasses: (1) human functioning (i.e. behaviour, cognition, emotion and motivation; and (2) human development, adaption, and change (i.e. personality/temperament, attachment, social systems and culture). Depending on the social work practice setting, different aspects of these bodies of knowledge from psychology will be emphasised. What is common across all contexts is the social work focus of considering a person in their environment (Kondrat, 2008). According to the Australian Association of Social Workers (2015, p. 4) the psychological aspects of a psychosocial assessment are informed by ecological, systems, and life-course theories. This means that people are best understood as relational beings, and as Sayer (2011, p. 119) suggests, 'individual agency develops through relationality and difference; what we are is dependent on but irreducible to such relations.'

Thus, social work tends to situate attention to psychological states, in assessments as individual responses to environmental events or pressures. Hutchison (2019) suggests that life-course theories, based on a range of empirical and theoretical work on the person-in-environment, utilise five main concepts in a biopsychosocial assessment: cohort, transitions, trajectories, life events, and turning points. *Cohorts* refers to the effect of historical events on people. For example, we could say that young people who were due to finish year 11 and 12 in Australia across 2020–2021 would be a cohort affected by the COVID-19 pandemic and the effects of this event are yet to emerge for this group. In life course theory, *transitions* refers to moments of stress and opportunity. Hutchison (2019, p. 353) suggests that births, marriages, divorce; remarriages, and deaths are considered to be transitions but increasingly the concept of transition can be applied to any changes to life course patterns which might contribute to stress. The concept of *trajectories* in life-course theory are used to consider patterns of life that are stable over the long term and 'are best understood in the rear-view mirror; the multiple transitions of a trajectory are usually not anticipated at earlier points along the life course' (Hutchison, 2019, p. 354).

Social workers using life-course theory would consider *life events* as significant events in a person's life that have impacted the functioning of an individual. These might include: parental divorce; ill-health or disability, experiences of violence or abuse; loss of community; experiences of disaster; and other major events. Lastly, Hutchison (2019, pp. 354–355) discusses the role of *turning points* as events that changed the course of the trajectory of a person, family, group, system or community. Myers (2016, p. 430) captures the sense of these turning points in her work with recovery stories in the field of mental health. They can be described after the Aristotelian concept of *peripeteia* where they constitute a 'breach' of life plan, followed by a subsequent erosion of moral agency and sense of connection to others. This description by Myers helps illuminate the connections between expressions of individual agency and autonomy and the social and cultural milieu in which they occur.

In these examples psychological states and experiences are intimately connected to social context and experience. One's psychological wellbeing and needs require understanding (e.g. assessment) and response (e.g. intervention) that is grounded in a person-in-environment thinking and a social justice ethic.

What Does the *Social* in a Bio-Psycho-Social-Spiritual Assessment Refer to?

From a social work perspective, the social has two main elements to it: the structural and the relational. Lawson and Garrod (2001, p. 494) explain that 'social structures are relatively permanent features of society that take on new characteristics different from the individuals who make up the social structure'. Some examples of social structures are the family, education, the law and work systems. Understanding that such systems exist, and that they have a history and can be impactful on much human behaviour is part of the social work knowledge repertoire. When social workers use a systems or ecological framework they will have these social structures in their minds as they undertake assessments (Australian Association of Social Workers, 2015).

Another structural aspect described by anti-oppressive social work perspectives (AOPs) is that of social divisions such as gender, class, race, ethnicity, sexual orientation and able-bodiedness (Thompson, cited in Hodgson & Watts, 2017, p. 84). AOP perspectives offer social workers intimate knowledge of discrimination, stigma and oppression. This knowledge is also an essential component of a social work perspective. These social divisions relate directly to the stress load many people carry that may affect their health, their capabilities and ability to live a good, non-humiliating life. It is well established that domination and discrimination contribute to the allostatic (stress) load many people carry (Johner, 2007). Social hierarchies have been demonstrated to have pernicious health effects; this has become known as the social gradient of health (Blane, 2005).

The second element of the social in any bio-psycho-social-spiritual perspective is *relational*. Relational refers to the insight that individuality is an emergent property from our embeddedness in social relations, beginning in infancy and continuing throughout our life (Donati & Archer, 2015). Charles Taylor (cited Sayer, 2011, p. 120) points to this relation when he says:

> one cannot be a self on one's own. I am a self only in relation to certain interlocutors: in one way in relation to those conversation partners who were essential to my achieving self-definition; in another in relation to those who are now crucial to my continuing grasp of languages and self-understanding.

It is from this relationship between ourselves and others that human agency is born – in the space between us. This is why social workers ask people about their families, their relationships and the general state of their social connections. They do this because this is a source of information about the web of relations that human beings require in order to support them when they are suffering, and to assist them to move towards a more flourishing life. Social workers also critique the political and social arrangements that undermine relations of care, as these relations are crucial for the meeting of human needs, dependencies, attachments and commitments. For example, social workers might critique and seek to address the lack of affordable housing or dangerous working conditions that affect the ability of families to meet basic needs.

What Does the *Spiritual* in a Bio-Psycho-Social-Spiritual Assessment Refer to?

There has been increasing attention in the literature of the spiritual side of human experience and what this means for social work theory and practice (Canda & Furman, 2009; Crisp, 2010; Hodgson & Watts, 2017; Holloway & Moss, 2010). Although sometimes linked, spirituality is conceptually distinct from religion and concerns 'existential questions of meaning, purpose, and how these relate to well-being, resilience, and healing' (Hodgson & Watts, 2017, p. 144). Canda and Furman (2009, p. 75, original italics) define spiritually as:

A process of human life and development:

- focussing on the search for a sense of meaning, purpose, morality and well-being;
- *in relationship* with oneself, other people, other beings, the universe, and ultimate reality however understood (e.g. in animistic, atheistic, nontheistic, polytheistic, theistic, or other ways);
- orienting around centrally significant priorities; and

- engaging in a sense of transcendence (experienced as deeply profound, sacred or transpersonal).

Much of the writing on spiritual assessment and practice in social work is in the context of palliative and oncology social work, as well as in mental health, disability, and chronic illness (e.g. Canda, 2009; Hodge, 2004; Reese, 2011; Stewart, 2014). This is because questions of hope, meaning, purpose, faith and transcendental experience can be particularly poignant in the context of dealing with health concerns, making major life adjustments, and facing one's mortality. As stated by Reese (2011, p. 204):

> The biopsychosocial-spiritual model looks at the spiritual history of a patient, whether religious or not, to add shape to his or her holistic identity. Illness strikes the whole person; interventions therefore focus on the biological, psychological, social, and spiritual dimensions.

Writers in the Unites States in particular have taken this further to develop specific tools and assessment questions that can help the social worker explore a person's spiritual beliefs and experiences (see for example, Nelson-Becker, Canda & Nakashima, 2016; Puchalski, 2006). Puchalski (2006) outlines a framework for a spiritual history, which includes: exploring faith and belief; its importance in the person's life; whether or not they belong to a faith community; and, the implication for health care and treatment. Nelson-Becker et al. (2016, pp. 77–78) propose eleven domains for exploration in spiritual assessment: spiritual affiliation, spiritual beliefs, spiritual behaviours, emotional qualities of spirituality; values; spiritual experiences; spiritual history; therapeutic change factors; social support, spiritual well-being; and, extrinsic/intrinsic spiritual focus. Hodge (cited in Stewart, 2014, p. 61) proposes some brief questions that may help the social worker explore and assess spiritual needs. These questions *may* be applicable in many health contexts, but care and discretion is needed in deciding *when* and how to explore such questions:

1 I was wondering if spirituality or religion is important to you?
2 Are there certain spiritual beliefs and practices that you find particularly helpful in dealing with problems?
3 I was also wondering if you attend a church or some other type of spiritual community?
4 Are there any spiritual needs or concerns I can help you with?

There is a relationship between spirituality and social justice. Hodge (2012) argues that spiritual worldviews are imbued with moral and ontological presuppositions, which provide guidance over matters of fairness, moral desert, right and wrong, and how the world is and how it ought to be. Such matters can aid in collaboratively identifying and responding to situations of injustice. Dylan and Coates (2012) posit that progressive eco-spirituality can act as a counterpoint to the destructive forces of modernity and resultant capitalism and neoliberalism, holding potential for ways of living and being that are more ecologically harmonious. In other word, the spiritual aspect of human experience is not only existentially important: it helps us surface broader questions about what kind of society we want to live in.

Reflection: Sharon's Story

Jack (47) and Sharon (42) live on the outskirts of a regional town in Western Australia with their seven children: Tom (15), Kevin (13), Jenny (12), Brooke (10), Jess (7) Georgie (6) and Marky (5). Jack and Sharon, moved the family to the area because they could find a cheaper place to live in a farmhouse attached to Jack's work as a farm labourer. Sharon, stayed at home to care for the family. Neither Jack nor Sharon have contact with their own parents or siblings.

Two years ago, Jack was injured in a farm accident leaving him permanently incapacitated from undertaking labouring work. As a result, the family had to move from their rented farmhouse into town where Sharon went to work shifts at the local abattoir, the only place she could get work as she had left school very early. The children had to move schools as part of the move into the town. The family have struggled to adjust to the changes, there was little money as the accident had not been covered sufficiently by insurance. Jack is not eligible for a Disability Support Pension and is not well enough to look for work either.

As the family adjusts to the changes, Jack begins drinking more and more and he becomes mean and difficult. With Sharon effectively out of the house working most of the time, Brooke and her older sister Jenny start to do most of the cooking and washing for the family, in addition to caring for the younger siblings, Jess, Georgie and Marky – including getting them to school. Most often Sharon is working or asleep when they have to leave for school. Jack is also frequently asleep in the mornings. Sharon is struggling to keep up with work and the family, compounded by frequent asthma and respiratory problems, which seem to affect the children as well.

One evening an argument breaks out between Jack and the older boys, which involved a lot of shouting and swearing. Sharon was home at the time and tried to intervene, but she had an asthma attack that could not be calmed down. A neighbour calls the police due to the noise and the police call an ambulance for Sharon. When Sharon is taken to hospital she is visibly distraught and sobbing uncontrollably and says she needs to go home immediately to look after the children. She also says she is exhausted from not sleeping and is worried the family are about to be evicted from their rental property because they are struggling to pay their rent on time.

Reflection Questions

1. What social justice concerns do you identify in Sharon's story?
2. What biological health issues or needs do you identify with Sharon and her family?
3. What sorts of things would help Sharon with her psychological wellbeing? As a social worker, how would you assess for this, and what sorts of things do you think are important to pay attention to here?
4. Identify a range of social needs that you feel could make a positive difference in the lives of Sharon and her family? In what ways might these address questions of social justice?
5. How might you approach a conversation with Sharon to understand more about the spiritual side of her experience? Importantly, *would* you approach this? Why or why not?

Conclusion

Social justice is a central value for social work and a guiding ideal that gives social work its purpose and its form. This chapter has linked a social justice perspective to the theoretical concepts that underpin the bio-psycho-social-spiritual dimensions of human experience. Social workers will frequently use a bio-psycho-social-spiritual framework in their assessments with service users in health settings. The purpose of this chapter has been to take a step back to explore the underpinning and informing ideas that help social workers connect assessment processes to the wider project of social justice. That is to say, a bio-psycho-social-spiritual perspective draws together a holistic and person-in-environment perspective of human health needs, and one that can help social workers collaborate with service users in ways that seek to address various injustices that impact on health and wellbeing.

Key Website Resources

AASW Scope of Practice: Psychosocial Assessments (www.aasw.asn.au/document/item/8312). This is the Australian Association of Social Workers psychosocial assessments scope of practice. It details what a psychosocial assessment is, and how and why social workers use this in their practice.

World Health Organization. (2021). First Global Conference – The Ottawa Charter World Health Organization (www.who.int/teams/health-promotion/enhanced-wellbeing/first-global-conference). This webpage offers the background to the first conference about public health and from which the Ottawa Charter emerged.

Edelman, C. L & Lush, E. (Hosts). (2021, October 1). The good news about the bad news about the global goals [Audio podcast episode] (https://globalgoalscast.org/s6e1). This is a podcast that offers stories from around the world about initiatives for progressing the UN Sustainable Development Goals (SDGs). The podcast has also covered the impact of the Global Pandemic on the progress of the SDGs. Each episode ends with what listeners can do to make a difference in their own communities.

References

Archer, M. S. (2007). *Making our way through the world: Human reflexivity and social mobility*. Cambridge, UK: Cambridge University Press.

Australian Association of Social Workers. (2015). Scope of social work practice: Psychosocial assessments. Retrieved from www.aasw.asn.au/document/item/8312.

Australian Association of Social Workers. (2020). Code of ethics. Retrieved from www.aasw.asn.au/document/item/13400.

Blane, D. (2005). The life course, the social gradient, and health. In M. Marmot & R. Wilkinson (eds), *Social determinants of health* (2nd edn., pp. 54–78). Oxford: Oxford University Press.

British Association of Social Workers. (2012). *The code of ethics for social work*. Retrieved from http://cdn.basw.co.uk/upload/basw_112315-7.pdf.

Canda, E. R. (2009). Chronic illness and transilience along my spiritual path. In D. Saleeby (ed.), *The strengths perspective in social work practice* (5th ed., pp. 72–92). New York: Pearson Education.

Canda, E. R. & Furman, L. D. (2009). *Spiritual diversity in social work practice: The heart of helping*. New York: Oxford University Press.

Corning, P. (2005). *Holistic Darwinism: Synergy, cybernetics, and the bioeconomics of evolution*. Chicago, IL: University of Chicago Press.

Crisp, B. R. (2010). *Spirituality and social work*. Farnham: Ashgate.

Donati, P. & Archer, M. S. (2015). *The relational subject*Cambridge: Cambridge University Press.

Doyal, M. & Gough, I. (1991). *A theory of human need*. New York: Guildford Press.

Dylan, A. & Coates, J. (2012). The spirituality of justice: Bringing together the eco and the social. *Journal of Religion & Spirituality in Social Work*, 31(1–2),128–149.

Hodge, D. R. (2004). Spirituality and people with mental illness: Developing spiritual competency in assessment and intervention. *Families in Society*, 85(1), 36–44. doi:10.1606/1044-3894.257.

Hodge, D. R. (2012). The conceptual and empirical relationship between spirituality and social justice: Exemplars from diverse faith traditions. *Journal of Religion & Spirituality in Social Work*, 31(1–2),32–50.

Hodgson, D. & Watts, L. (2017). *Key concepts and theory in social work*. London: Palgrave Macmillan.

Holloway, M. & Moss, B. (2010). *Spirituality and social work*. Basingstoke: Palgrave Macmillan.

Hunt, J. (2014). Bio-psycho-social-spiritual assessment? Teaching the skill of spiritual assessment. *Social Work and Christianity*, 41(4), 373.

Hutchison, E. D. (2019). An update on the relevance of the life course perspective for social work. *Families in Society: The Journal of Contemporary Social Services*, 100(4), 351–366. doi:10.1177/1044389419873240.

Johner, R. L. (2007). Allostatic load: Single parents, stress-related health issues, and social care. *Health & Social Work*, 32(2), 89–94. doi:10.1093/hsw/32.2.89.

Kondrat, M. E. (2008). Person-in-environment. In T. Mizrahi & L. E. Davis (ed.), *Encyclopaedia of social work* (20th edn., pp. 348–354). NASW Press.

Lawson, T. & Garrod, J. (2001). *Dictionary of sociology*. Taylor & Francis Group.

Marmot, M. (2005). Social determinants of health inequalities. *The Lancet*, 365(9464), 1099–1104. doi:10.1016/S0140-6736(05)71146-71146.

Marmot, M., Friel, S., Bell, R., Houweling, T. A. J. & Taylor, S. (2008). Closing the gap in a generation: health equity through action on the social determinants of health. *The Lancet*, 372 (9650), 1661–1669. doi:10.1016/S0140-6736(08)61690-61696.

McKay, F. H. & Taket, A. (2020). *Health equity, social justice, and human rights* (2nd ed.). Routledge.

Myers, N. A. L. (2016). Recovery stories: An anthropological exploration of moral agency in stories of mental health recovery. *Transcultural Psychiatry*, 53(4), 427–444. doi:10.1177/1363461516663124.

National Association of Social Workers. (2015). Code of ethics. Retrieved from www.socialworkers.org/pubs/code/.

Nelson-Becker, H., Canda, E. R. & Nakashima, M. (2016). Spirtuality in professional practice with older adults. In D. B. Kaplan & B. Berkman (eds), *The Oxford handbook of social work in health and aging* (2nd edn., pp. 73–84). New York: Oxford University Press.

Puchalski, C. (2006). Spiritual assessment in clinical practice. *Psychiatric Annals*, 36(3), 150–155. doi:10.3928/00485713-20060301-06.

Reese, D. (2011). Spirtuality and social work practice in palliative care. In T. Altilio & S. Otis-Green (eds), *Oxford textbook of palliative social work* (pp. 201–213). New York: Oxford University Press.

Sayer, R. A. (2011). *Why things matter to people: Social science, values and ethical life*: Cambridge: Cambridge University Press.

Sen, A. (2002). Why health equity? *Health Economics*, 11(8), 659–666. doi:10.1002/hec.762.

Stewart, M. (2014). Spiritual assessment: A patient-centered approach to oncology social work practice. *Social Work in Health Care*, 53(1), 59–73. doi:10.1080/00981389.2013.834033.

Venkatapuram, S. (2011). *Health justice: An argument from the capabilities approach*. Cambridge: Polity Press.

Watts, L. & Hodgson, D. (2019). *Social justice theory and practice for social work: Critical and philosophical perspectives*. Singapore: Springer.

World Health Organization. (1986). The Ottowa charter for health promotion. Retrieved from www.who.int/healthpromotion/conferences/previous/ottawa/en/index1.html.

Young, I. M. (1990). *Justice and the politics of difference*. Princeton, NJ: Princeton University Press.

3 Neoliberal Capitalism and its Impact on Individual and Community Health

Implications for Critical Social Workers

Niki Edwards and Julie King

Introduction

Social work is a contributor to the Australian health care system; practitioners are active across the human lifespan and the health care continuum. Regardless of where social workers practice, health will be of key importance to individuals, their human and environmental relationships and contexts. Improvements to the health of Australians and the global citizenship requires critical insights and knowledge of the determinants of health to ensure interventions are appropriate and socially just. To do this, neoliberalism requires close examination given the capitalist ideology connects political, economic and social institutions to health.

Criticisms of the impacts of neoliberalism on health and healthcare services are not new. About 40 years ago the radical Welsh general practitioner, epidemiologist and social advocate, Julian Tudor Hart introduced the inverse care law; arguing that availability of good medical care tended to vary inversely with the need for the population served (and this) operated more so when medical care was most exposed to market forces (Hart, 1971). Until his death in 2018, he was tireless in his critique of capitalism and its negative consequences on health.

He is not alone in his sentiments; Nicky Hart, USA professor of sociology and health inequalities researcher, reviewed a health text that understood ill-health resulting from the social and economic organisation of society, *The Political Economy of Health* (Doyal, 1979). Hart provocatively titled her review 'Is capitalism bad for your health?'. In it she discussed significant improvements in mortality that had followed societal transformation arising from post industrialisation conditions of living (Hart, 1982). However, Hart concurred with the premise of Doyal (1979) there were inherent contradictions in health progress as some individuals benefitted but other people and communities remained 'spectacularly' disadvantaged, and in fact, at increased risk. Almost a decade later, Vincente Navarro, Spanish sociologist and political scientist published his text *Dangerous to Your Health: Capitalism in Health Care* (Navarro, 1993). He posited that access to healthcare reforms were necessitated to ensure the human right to health. So, what has changed?

In 2012, Australian health economist and advocate of social justice in healthcare Gavin Mooney (2012) similarly titled his article, 'Neoliberalism is bad for our health'. More recently Ted Schrecker, a UK-based political scientist, published (with his colleague) *How Politics Makes Us Sick: Neoliberal Epidemics* (Schrecker & Bambra, 2015). Waitzkin (2020), an activist physician and professor of sociology in the USA, summed up what needed to shift when he released his article, 'Moving beyond capitalism for our health.'

DOI: 10.4324/9781003330745-4

Some consider capitalism under neoliberalism to be a form of structural violence that disproportionately affects the most vulnerable of the population (Sakellariou & Rotarou, 2017); and others implicate neoliberalism in the rise and persistence of health inequalities (Collins et al., 2015). Neoliberalism is a political determinant of health, sitting alongside the social and commercial determinants (Viens, 2019; Flynn, 2021). This chapter argues the importance of social workers adopting a social model of health; specifically use of a 'social lens' of health. This is imperative given that capitalist governments around the globe, including the Australian government, have 'shirked' societal level population health responsibilities through an express focus on individual responsibility for health. Neoliberalism is a driver of health inequalities; hence there are obligations for critical social workers who seek social justice and human rights through anti-oppressive practice. Social workers can bridge professional practice at micro and meso levels to advocate for macro level, systemic changes that embrace and respond to the social, commercial and political determinants of health that are ignored and neglected by neoliberalism.

Neoliberalism

Neoliberalism is a somewhat confusing inherently conservative concept (Eliason, 2015) but is typically understood as 'the' way society is organised and few recognise alternatives. It is the primary ideology driving governments, economy, and contemporary healthcare delivery. Historical roots can be traced back to liberalism as conceptualised by Adam Smith as published in *The Wealth of Nations* in the middle of the eighteenth century. After the Second World War, the welfare state emerged side-by-side with government management of the economy (Chapman, 2016). At this time the concept of 'citizenship' was important where all members of society regardless of income or productivity were entitled to essential services inclusive of health and other welfare requirements (Merone & Ashton, 2021). However, the economist and philosopher Hayek was very influential (Freeman, 2018). He believed economies were too complex for governments beckoning in an era characterised by free markets, free trade, strong property rights and minimal government interference (Hayek, 1944). Modern neoliberalism emerged as a global force in the 1980s, driven by policies implemented by the International Monetary Fund, the World Bank and the United States Treasury Department to aid countries in crisis; known as the Washington Consensus (Sakellariou & Rotarou, 2017). Neoliberalism has arisen from distaste of state-planned economies that were conceptualised as autocratic and repressive of individual liberties (Baum et al., 2016). This political 'capitalist' ideology has dominated much of the industrialised world for a number of centuries.

Neoliberalism has been considered as a 'sloppy' synonym for capitalism (Ferguson, 2010) and 'super-capitalism' because of its reliance on an intensely competitive market that is unregulated and dependent on consumerism (Chapman, 2016). Despite numerous economic, social, political, and philosophical definitions, there are three key and influential tenets: individualism, privatisation, and decentralisation (McGregor, 2001). At the ideological heart as Hayek theorised, is the competitive and private free market, reduced public expenditure on infrastructure and services, and deregulation that is understood to enable freedom of choice and economic activities. There is significant emphasis placed on deregulation, minimalisation of the state, privatisation, commodification and individual responsibility (Huber & Niedzwiecki, 2018; Viens, 2019). Individual responsibility is important to recognise when focusing on health and wellbeing; neoliberalism encompasses both economic theory and normative ideals of self and society (Roberts, 2020). Such values shape delivery of health policy and services, including notion that health is an economic good. Many contemporary health and health care discourses are informed by liberal capitalism, given that this has been an era that has seen inherent assumptions become less an idea than an orthodoxy (Cheek, 2008).

Most societies in the Global North accept neoliberalist capitalism as the 'norm'; rhetoric of this hegemonic ideological project is linked to political freedom and hence the logic argues, healthy societies (Baru and Mohan, 2018). While Barnett and Bagshaw (2020) suggested neoliberalism 'swallowed' the world they caution against such acceptance. Critical exploration of alternatives is required given neoliberalism has far reaching impacts on political, cultural and social processes, and this includes health. (Mudge, 2008). Further, neoliberalism is embedded within strategically powerful global institutions including the World Bank, the United Nations (UN) and the World Health Organization (WHO) that all prioritise addressing health inequalities and the intersection with poverty, and disadvantage. Nonetheless, these global organisations have failed to act decisively, and progress has been slow (Mooney, 2012). There is growing evidence of negative impacts of neoliberalism on healthcare; use of economic policies such as austerity have had a devastating effect on health equity (Viens, 2019).

Reflection Questions

- Is health a human right? In Australia? In the Global South?
- How is health and wellbeing understood and realised within neoliberal societies?
- How can individual responsibility for health and wellbeing (healthism) be challenged?

Neoliberalism and Health

'Health' is understood by most people as a fundamental human right. However, neoliberalism considers health as a particular kind of economic good; as a commodity governed by market principles (Viens, 2019). Health and health care in this neoliberal climate is a tradeable commodity rather than a collective good or human right; and further, an individual responsibility (Bell & Green, 2016). Health services are hence professionally structured in a way to maximise instrumental value. Neoliberal healthcare systems value a free competitive market, considering this approach most cost-effective (Merone & Ashton, 2021). This might be through production of efficient and innovative care, comparable with how health services are structured under a welfare system.

Health becomes a negatively defined value (i.e. absence of disease), which encourages a problem of overstating healthcare as a determinant of health with market-based responses that focus on remediation (Braveman, 2014). Neither considered a special or unique human experience, health is an instrumental good traded-off with other needs (Baum et al., 2016). In Australia, Baum et al. (2016) note the discernible public sector trend towards a market-oriented discourse of health services management, in which the collective good of health is ignored, and violations of this human right directly contributes to health inequalities. Of significant concern, the current Australian government appears to have moved away from the ethical and moral responsibilities for health of all citizens through adoption of the individual responsibility mantra (i.e. the individualisation of health).

Defining Health: Tensions with Reductionism

Few would argue that health, ill-health and disease cannot be simply reduced down to biological phenomena. Limits of reductionist approaches to health were acknowledged by the WHO in 1948 when health was defined as a state of complete physical, mental and social well-being and not merely the absence of disease or infirmity (World Health Organization, 1948). This often-quoted definition implies a range of biological, psychological and social factors influence health. Furthermore, health is conceptualised as not merely the absence of disease, but rather in the positive sense of well-being. While this definition has been criticised for its utopian and vague notions of 'complete well-being', it is of symbolic importance because it highlights need for a broader approach to health than the biomedical model alone (Germov, 2019).

The WHO definition of health has not been amended since inception after the Second World War and it remains highly persuasive and in popular use globally. There are positive attributes, including:

- Consistent with the biopsychosocial model of health.
- Considers physiological, psychological and social factors in health and illness, and interactions between factors.
- Attention to holistic nature of health e.g. ecosystem perspective.
- Inclusive of context of everyday life environments.
- Multidimensional and acknowledges multiplicity of factors.
- Positive approach.

However, despite being considered innovative and even somewhat revolutionary initially, perhaps the definition and understanding of health needs revision? There are serious criticisms relevant for critical social workers working in the health space. These include (Dodge et al., 2012):

- Too broad: how many people have complete physical, mental and social wellbeing all the time? What does complete mean?
- Pathologisation of life: does this view of health contribute to medicalisation of society? Medicalisation of less than perfect health status?
- One size fits all: does not embrace temporary 'ill health', chronic illness or disability? If a person lives with chronic illness, impairment or disability, are they unable to be 'healthy'?
- An identity claim: you are not truly healthy unless you are *totally* healthy.
- Idealistic: not realistic and never achievable? Hence, most people unhealthy most of the time?
- Value-laden: needs objective, scientific inspection and measurement?

The definition is also devoid of cultural diversity; failing to recognise or respond to different ways of understanding health and illness. While the definition clearly does has positive attributes, it is very individualistic and take little account of the broader social, commercial and political determinants of health. It neglects to iterate health as a human right and ignores any collective responsibility or social mandates.

Huber and his colleagues in the Netherlands have argued for an alternative to the WHO definition, suggesting it is no longer fit for its purpose (Huber et al., 2011). They proposed a new definition of health as 'the ability to adapt and to self-manage in the face of social, physical and emotional challenges'. Their definition captures health as having a number of dynamic features and dimensions. Huber et al. (2011) argued focus should be on the ability of people to adapt to their situations as key to health; this social lens of health is consistent with the biopsychosocial/ spiritual/cultural or ecological person-in-environment approach adopted by social workers. Their definition acknowledges that health is subjective in so far that personal meanings and embedded experiences will differ between people and societies, with linkages to context and particular needs.

Nonetheless, both the WHO and the Huber et al. definitions place considerable heavy obligations on the individual who is still held responsible for health status. Emphasis on lifestyle diseases pervades such expectations. Mortality and morbidity have been linked to lifestyle-related risk factors (Crosland et al., 2019). These factors are considered largely preventable: smoking/tobacco use, alcohol consumption, high body mass index, physical inactivity and a poor diet. There are obvious impacts of the design and delivery of healthcare services given that approximately one third of the health burden in Australia is attributable to modifiable risk factors. However, this is far too simplistic, assumes individuals are the locus of control, and there is no doubt there is a very unequal distribution of toxic experiences that shape health and wellbeing (Baciu et al., 2017).

Healthism: 'If You Get Sick, it is Your Fault'

Most people doggedly believe they control their own personal choices and ultimately destiny inclusive of health status. Regardless, missing is deep awareness that an individual is *not* solely responsible for their health and wellbeing status. People and communities are influenced by the complex interplay of culture, customs, and social institutions that scaffold life and wellbeing. This discriminatory view that the individual holds full responsibility for their health and wellbeing is called 'healthism'. Healthism is a phenomenon that first emerged during the 1980s; joining other 'isms' such as racism, ageism or ableism. Crawford (1980), an economist, described it as preoccupation with personal health as a primary focus for the definition and achievement of well-being; the goal was obviously attained lifestyle modification. However, healthism was first described by Zola (1977), a sociologist who examined the impacts of medicalisation on society and saw individual responsibility for health as producing highly undesirable side-effects. Healthism was also about social control, specifically about what people should and should not do within their lived experiences, in order to be 'healthy'. There were medical and social expectations at play.

Neoliberalism positions and conceptualises health as the property and responsibility of the individual. Personal pursuit of health is prioritised above anything else in order to be a productive 'good' citizen. Naturally solutions and strategies are also posed at the individual level (Zola, 1977). There is no acknowledgement of the complex social milieu that people live within, the consequences of physical and social environments, or impacts of time or history. Informed by healthism, health status should be widely recognised as an anti-discrimination category. Critical social workers might argue that discrimination linked to health is akin to race, religion, gender, sexual orientation, disability or age (Roberts & Weeks, 2016).

Human-created, social aspects of life are highly influential on health and this is in direct contrast with purely random events or products of nature (López & Scott, 2000). This awareness is not new as Marx and Engels connected links between disease, and poor living and working conditions as an outcome of capitalist exploitation (Germov, 2019). Germov (2019) notes that Engels highlighted differences in death rates between labourers and professionals, claiming that the squalid living conditions of the working class were primarily responsible for the disparity. While the 'social' in medicine held sway at different points in history, there have been significant changes to healthcare; doctors and other healthcare professionals must now vie for market share and power in the neoliberal market; influencing how health is conceptualised and managed in the twenty-first century (Timmermans & Oh, 2010). Although the biomedical model remains dominant, a major criticism is that this reductionism underestimates the complexity of health and illness; specifically neglecting the intersectionality of the social, commercial and political determinants that Engels identified as being linked to post-industrial society generated capitalism. Hart spoke to this in his 1971 article when he introduced the inverse care law; many scholars and clinicians remain concerned about how the broader wellbeing of societies around the world have been eroded by the negative health impacts of neoliberalism.

Social inequality has a central impact on ability of people and populations to be healthy; social and environmental factors rather than individual factors are *most* influential. Despite this reality, neoliberal governments, including the Australian government is guilty of healthism by dogmatically pursuing notions of individual autonomy and promotion of individual responsibility. Such an approach negates and obscures state ethical and moral responsibilities to protect and promote the wellbeing of all Australian citizens. This neglect continues despite a growing body of evidence about the importance of structural determinants of health, especially the role of political and commercial determinants of health at the national and global levels (Viens, 2019). Health needs to be understood outside of the capitalist lens with its focus on economic determinants (e.g. far more than an economic good governed by market forces). Simply, individuals cannot freely exercise 'choices' around health. The hegemony of neoliberal ideology pervades how global citizens understand health, how healthcare should be structured, and how to respond to ill-health and related health issues.

Social Model of Health: Health through a Social Lens

If people are questioned about what determines their health and wellbeing, they are unlikely to be aware of the social or commercial determinants of health (see Chapter 1). They are much more likely to identify and discuss the primacy of biomedical elements that influence their choices and hence behaviours. The social model of health goes beyond the social, commercial and political determinants of health (Germov, 2019); it has been around for decades and is a general umbrella term that captures approaches that focus on the social determinants of health and illness (Broom 1991). This social lens of health does not erase or replace the biomedical model; it extends important dimensions that are of consequence and influence.

Structural barriers to health and healthcare often stem from uncomfortable forces of oppression like racism, sexism, classism, and heterosexism. There are hence moral and ethical obligations to address the whole person, and social workers are well aware that each person makes individual choices regarding their health *but* they are embedded in families, neighbourhoods, and societies. All of those levels contain factors of dynamic influence on individual opportunities, choices and behaviour; whether that behaviour is smoking, nutritional patterns, physical activity, or meditating (Eliason, 2015). However, health interventions or health promotion typically targets diet, physical activity, smoking and alcohol consumption. Recommended changes in lifestyle choices are underpinned by moral imperatives linked to healthism (e.g. often social consequences for those people who are deemed less worthy than others or stigmatised and discriminated against). 'You are what you eat' comes to mind but when there is reflection around the nexus between race or ethnicity, poverty, unstable income, inability to access food required for good nutrition and geographical isolation; individual choice becomes highly problematic.

This model argues that many illnesses and health problems are socially produced and go beyond the control of individuals (Germov, 2019). A social lens of health and well-being scrutinises the role that living and working conditions play in both contributing to or remedying health and illness. The key dimensions (Table 3.1) are provided below; the need for co-development with individuals and communities, cultural safety and respectful bottom-up approaches are obvious. Using a social model of health, critical social workers must work towards equitable healthcare by embracing cultural safety and critical consciousness; this involves critiquing power structures as well as challenging their own privilege and culture as opposed to looking to be 'competent' with regards to other cultures (Curtis et al., 2019). This a process of embracing the richness of cultural and linguistic differences and decolonising practice. Relevance and importance in healthcare has been welcomed by Aboriginal and Torres Strait Islander peoples who experience significant health gaps and disparities (Bennett & Gates, 2019) but relevance goes beyond healthcare services for Indigenous peoples (see Chapter 12).

Table 3.1 Key dimensions of the social lens of health

1.	Individual health is enabled or inhibited by the broader social, cultural, economic and political context. While individual voice, agency and choices can play critical roles (e.g. lifestyle choices); the socio-cultural context people live and work within play powerful influences on health and ill-health.
2.	The human body is simultaneously social, psychological, spiritual, cultural and biological. It is much more than simply biology, physiology and anatomy.
3.	Health is political, crossing and overlapping private and public domains of life. Political processes have a significant influence. It is important to recognise the intersection of the social, commercial and political determinants of health.
3.	Health is cultural; ways in which health is perceived and experienced are expressed vary from culture to culture and within cultures. Cultural safety is imperative; involving an environment promoting health and wellbeing while simultaneously spiritually, socially, emotionally and physically safe for all people. This trauma-informed approach welcomes people and works within communities in regard to who they are and what they need. There is celebration of identity as opposed to assault, challenge or denial.
4.	Biomedicine and medical science can provide and contribute to health and ill-health but are part of requirements. Embracing holistic approaches to wellbeing implicates need for socio-psycho-social-spiritual-cultural-biomedical engagement, assessment and interventions. Importance of person-in-environment (ecological) approaches is acknowledged, inclusive of the social *and* physical environment.
5.	Agency and voices matter: it is imperative to respond to voices of people outside of medicine. The person/patient/client is the expert in their own lives. This expertise should be sought, deeply listened to, respected and privileged.

Source: informed by Yuill, Crinson and Duncan (2010)

Human Rights, Health and Neoliberalism: The Challenges

Neoliberalism proposes that every part of human life can be commodified and exploited for economic gain, as is the case for health (Esposito & Perez, 2014; MacNaughton & Frey, 2018). However, this approach means that many people are deprived of their right to health. A human rights-based approach emphasises that every person has fundamental rights to health that should be respected and protected. All people have the right to the enjoyment of the highest attainable standard of health and to the surprise of many, such rights are actually protected by international law.

The right to health was first articulated in the WHO 1946 constitution as the highest attainable standard of health as a fundamental right of every human being; and the 1948 UN Universal Declaration of Human Rights states that everyone has the right to a standard of living adequate for health, including medical care and social services (Office of the United Nations High Commissioner for Human Rights, 1948). The 1948 Universal Declaration of Human Rights also mentions health as part of the right to an adequate standard of living (article 25). It was again recognised as a human right in 1966 in the International Covenant on Economic, Social and Cultural Rights (ICESCR) that Australia is a party to; noting Article 12:

1 The States Parties to the present Covenant recognize the right of everyone to the enjoyment of the highest attainable standard of physical and mental health.
2 The steps to be taken by the States Parties to the present Covenant to achieve the full realization of this right shall include those necessary for:
    a The provision for the reduction of the stillbirth-rate and of infant mortality and for the healthy development of the child;
    b The improvement of all aspects of environmental and industrial hygiene;
    c The prevention, treatment and control of epidemic, endemic, occupational and other diseases;
    d The creation of conditions which would assure to all medical service and medical attention in the event of sickness.

Australia is a party to seven core international human rights treaties that embrace the right to health, inclusive of the ICESCR. Also relevant is article 5(iv) of the Convention on the Elimination of All Forms of Racial Discrimination (CERD), articles 10(h), 11(1)(f), 12, 14 (2)(b) and 16(1)(e) of the Convention on the Elimination of All Forms of Discrimination Against Women (CEDAW), articles 24 and 25 of the Convention on the Rights of the Child (CRC) and articles 23(1)(c) and 25 of the Convention on the Rights of Persons with Disabilities (CRPD) (see www.ohchr.org/EN/HRBodies/Pages/TreatyBodies.aspx).

However, despite fundamentally global agreement on the right to health, Merone and Ashton (2021) reported that in 2011, only 25% of national constitutions across the globe guaranteed, or aspired to, the right to public health for all citizens. Amy Kapczynski, US professor of law points out the right to health that has been enshrined in some nations' legislation has led to a growing number of successful cases where individuals have 'won' the right to access to unaffordable medicine through legal action (Kapczynski, 2019). While such 'success' appears applaudable, she points out beneficiaries of these cases are disadvantaged individuals and the very poorest of patients remain deprived. Such approaches fail to recognise systemic barriers to healthcare that exist in the first place. Although the cases were successful, they reflect broader structural issues compromising rights to health: including, under-resourced and strained healthcare systems, relying on public funding and allowing pharmaceutical companies to continue overcharging for their products (Kapczynski, 2019). Kapczynski (2019) also cations that other systemic changes are required to redress structural drivers of health inequalities. Conventional healthcare rarely challenges fundamental, underlying structures that produce ill-health (Yamin, 2019).

Such experiences are relevant to Australian healthcare. It is highly likely that international law in general and human rights law will come to play increasingly important roles in healthcare delivery in the future (Broberg & Sanoo, 2017). For example, in Queensland, Australia, the Human Rights Act 2019 came into effect in January 2020. Consistent with Australia's international obligations, this legislation includes right to access health services without discrimination and stipulates a person must not be refused emergency life-saving treatment. This legislation provides an inextricable link between public health and human rights and will provide an avenue for litigation against breaches to rights to healthcare. Schetzer (2020) in reviewing the implementation of the Queensland Human Rights Act commented that the legislation fell short in providing effective, accessible remedies and causes of action for individuals who allege that their rights have been violated. She added that under international law, access to effective dispute resolution mechanisms and compensation was considered essential but was not provided. Health advocacy is a key role for critical social workers who need to work with lawyers to ensure social justice is achieved in this space as well.

Reflection Questions

- What are the social, commercial and political determinants of health? How do the commercial and political determinants of health differ from conditions in which people are born, grow, work, live and age?
- Why has neoliberalism reduced the comprehensiveness of healthcare and how have disadvantaged groups fared?
- What are the health impacts of the intersectionality of healthism and other oppressed identities including racism, gender, disability, poverty etc.?
- What can critical social workers do to reconcile micro and meso practice with the activism required at the macro level (i.e. how to redress systemic drivers of health inequalities)?

Conclusion

Social inequality has a pervasive impact on the ability of people and populations to be healthy, it is political action around these states of affairs that determines the extent of our success in the prevention and mitigation of ill health (Viens, 2019). Governments have a key role – linked to social, moral and ethical obligations – that goes far beyond neoliberal austerity policies and free market principles.

Calls for a new paradigm in understanding and redressing health problems is far from new (Siddique, 2018). The eminent sociologist C. Wright Mills (1916–1962) eloquently said that employment, war, marriage and problems of the city were public issues not just private issues. He thought individual solutions would never be sufficient to address lasting improvements for individuals *and* society. Mills described social scientists as those who ask imaginative questions, seeking answers beyond the obvious, searching for the obscure, and the unexpected answer (Mills, 1959). Critical social workers can be inspired to use creativity and their sociological imagination; to use social analysis to understand how capitalism negatively impacts the profession, clients and communities. The COVID-19 pandemic has affirmed social work as an essential profession given roles in addressing complex health crises arising (Ashcroft et al., 2021). The intersection of COVID-19, with the global impact of neoliberalism on the everyday responsibilities of critical social workers involved in healthcare delivery, highlights the fourfold impacts of capitalism: marketisation, consumerism, managerialism and de-professionalisation of social work (Ornellas et al., 2020).

Neoliberalism has an inherent disregard for a human-rights based approach to health that are enshrined in international law but ignored by capitalism; use of a 'social lens' of health is required if the core elements of a right to health: availability, accessibility and quality including safety, effectiveness, people-centeredness, timeliness, integration, efficiency and equity are to be realised by all citizens (Merone & Ashton, 2021). Neoliberal approaches that prioritise healthism (i.e. individual responsibility) need to be replaced by policies and services that reflect socially just community values. At minimum, critical social workers should carefully reflect and consider how their actions and inactions purposely address health inequalities informed by the social, commercial and political determinants of health. Neoliberalism is bad for your health!

References

Anderson, I. *et al.* (2016). Indigenous and tribal peoples' health (The Lancet–Lowitja Institute global collaboration): a population study, *Lancet*, 388(10040), 131–157.

Ashcroft, R. *et al.* (2021). The impact of the COVID-19 pandemic on social workers at the frontline: a survey of Canadian social workers, *The British Journal of Social Work*, 52(3), 1724–1746.

Baum, F. *et al.* (2016). Comprehensive primary health care under neo-liberalism in Australia, *Social Science & Medicine*, 168, 43–52.

Barnett, P and Bagshaw, P. (2020). Neoliberalism: what it is, how it affects health and what to do about it, *New Zealand Medical Journal*, 133(151), 76–84.

Baciu, A. *et al.* (2017). *Communities in Action: Pathways to Health Equity*, Washington, DC: National Academies Press.

Baru, R. & Mohan, M. (2018). Globalisation and neoliberalism as structural drivers of health inequities, *Health Research Policy Systems*, 16, 91.

Bell, K. & Green, J. (2016). On the perils of invoking neoliberalism in public health critique, *Critical Public Health*, 26(3), 239–243.

Bennett, B. & Gates, T. (2019). Teaching cultural humility for social workers serving LGBTQI Aboriginal communities in Australia, *Social Work Education*, 8(5), 604–617.

Booysen, F., Botha, F. & Wouters, E. (2021). Conceptual causal models of socioeconomic status, family structure, family functioning and their role in public health, *BMC Public Health*, 21(191),

Braveman, P. (2014). What are health disparities and health equity? We need to be clear, *Public Health Reports*, 129(Suppl 2), 5–8.

Braveman, P. & Gottlieb, L. (2014). The social determinants of health: it's time to consider the causes of the causes, *Public Health Reports*, 129 (Suppl 2), 19–31.

Broberg, M. & Sanoo, H. (2017). Strengths and weaknesses in a human rights-based approach to international development – an analysis of a rights-based approach to development assistance based on practical experiences, *The International Journal of Human Rights*, 22(5), 664–680.

Broom, D. (1991). *Damned if We Do: Contradictions in Women's Health Care.* London: Allen and Unwin.

Chapman, A. (2016). *Global Health, Human Rights, and the Challenge of Neoliberal Policies*, Cambridge: Cambridge University Press.

Cheek J. (2008). Healthism: a new conservatism? *Qualitative Health Research*, 18(7):974–982.

Collins, C., McCartney, G. & Garnham, L. (2015). Neoliberalism and health inequalities, in K. Smith, C. Bambra & S. Hill (eds), *Health Inequalities: Critical Perspectives*, Oxford Scholarship Online.

Coggon, J. & Viens, A. M. (2017). *Public Health Ethics in Practice*, London: Public Health England.

Crawford, R., (1980). Healthism and the medicalization of everyday life, *International Journal of Health Sciences*, 10(3), 365–388.

Crosland, P. *et al.* (2019). The health burden of preventable disease in Australia: a systematic review, *Australian and New Zealand Journal of Public Health*, 43(2), 163–170.

Curtis, E. *et al.* (2019). Why cultural safety rather than cultural competency is required to achieve health equity: a literature review and recommended definition, *International Journal for Equity in Health*, 18, 174.

de Lacy-Vawdon, C. & Livingstone, C. (2020). Defining the commercial determinants of health: a systematic review, *BMC Public Health*, 20, 1022.

Dodge, R., Daly, A., Huyton, J. & Sanders, L. (2012). The challenge of defining wellbeing. *International Journal of Wellbeing*, 2(3), 222–235. doi:10.5502/ijw.v2i3.4

Doyal, L. (1979). *The Political Economy of Health* (with I. Pennell), London: Pluto Press.

Eliason, M. (2015). Neoliberalism and health, *Advances in Nursing Science*, 38(1), 2–4.

Esposito, L. & Perez, F. M. (2014). Neoliberalism and the commodification of mental health, *Humanity & Society*, 38(4), 414–442.

Ferguson, J. (2010). The uses of neoliberalism, *Antipode*, 41(1), 166–184.

Flynn, M. (2021). Global capitalism as a societal determinant of health: a conceptual framework, *Social Science & Medicine*, 268(C).

Freeman, J. (2018). Reconsidering 'Set the people free': neoliberalism and freedom rhetoric in Churchill's Conservative Party, *Twentieth Century British History*, 29, 522–546.

Germov, J. (2019). Imagining health problems as social issues, In J. Germov (ed.), *Second Opinion: An Introduction to Health Sociology*, 6th edition, Melbourne: Oxford University Press.

Hart, J. (1971). The inverse care law, *Lancet*, 1, 405–412.

Hart, N. (1982). Review: is capitalism bad for your health? *The British Journal of Sociology*, 33(3), 435–443.

Hayek, F. (1944). *The Road to Serfdom*, George Routledge and Sons.

Huber, M. *et al.* (2011). How should we define health? *British Medical Journal*, 26(343): d4163.

Huber, E. & Niedzwiecki, S. (2018). Changing systems of social protection in the context of the changing political economies since the 1980s, *Cien Saude Colet*, 23(7), 2085–2094.

Kapczynski, A. (2019). The right to medicines in an age of neoliberalism, *Humanity: An International Journal of Human Rights, Humanitarianism, and Development*, 10(1), 79–107.

Kickbusch, I., Allen, L. & Franz, C. (2016). The commercial determinants of health, *Lancet Global Health*, 12, e895–e896.

Lang, T. & Rayner, G. (2012). Ecological public health: the 21st century's big idea, *British Medical Journal*, 345, e5466.

López, J. & Scott, J. (2000). *Social Structure*, Open University Press.

MacNaughton, G. & Frey, D. (2018). Challenging neoliberalism: ILO, human rights, and public health frameworks on decent work, *Health and Human Rights*, 20(2), 43.

McGregor, S., (2001). Neoliberalism and health care, *International Journal of Consumer Studies*, 25(2), 82–89.

Merone, L. & Ashton, S. (2021). The inextricable link between public health and human rights and threats to progression in far-right populism and neoliberal systems, *Australia and New Zealand Journal of Public Health*, 45(5), 417–419.

Mialon M. (2020). An overview of the commercial determinants of health, *Globalization and Health*, 16(1), 74.

Millar, J. (2013). The corporate determinants of health: how big business affects our health, and the need for government action, *Canadian Journal of Public Health*, 104(4), e327–e329.

Mills, C. (1959). *The Sociological Imagination*, London: Oxford University Press.

Mooney, G. (2012). Neoliberalism is bad for our health, *International Journal of Health Services* 42 (3):383–401.

Mudge, S. (2008). The state of the art: what is neoliberalism, *Socio-Economic Review*, 6, 703–733.

Navarro, V. (1993). *Dangerous to Your Health: Capitalism in Health Care*, New York Monthly Review Press.

Office of the United Nations High Commissioner for Human Rights. (1948). *The Universal Declaration of Human Rights*, Geneva: United Nations.

Ornellas, A, Engelbrecht, L & Atamtürk, E. (2020). The fourfold neoliberal impact on social work and why this matters in times of the COVID-19 pandemic and beyond, *Social Work*, 56(3), 235–249.

Roberts, M. (2020). Globalization and neoliberalism: structural determinants of global mental health? *Humanity and Society*, online first.

Roberts, J. & Weeks, E., (2016). What is (and isn't) healthism, *Georgia Law Review*, 50.

Sakellariou, D. & Rotarou, E. S. (2017). The effects of neoliberal policies on access to healthcare for people with disabilities, *International Journal for Equity in Health*, 16(1), 199.

Schetzer, L. (2020). Queensland's Human Rights Act: perhaps not such a great step forward, *Alternative Law Journal*, 45(1), 12–17.

Schrecker, T. & Bambra, C. (2015). *How Politics Makes Us Sick: Neoliberal Epidemics*, Basingstoke: Palgrave Macmillan.

Siddique, J. (2018). Toward a new paradigm of health and human potential, *World Futures*, 74(2), 116–133.

Spolander, G. *et al.* (2014). The implications of neoliberalism for social work: Reflections from a six-country international research collaboration, *International Social Work*, 57(4), 301–312.

Timmermans, S. & Oh, H. (2010). The continued social transformation of the medical profession, *Journal of Health and Social Behaviour*, 51, S94–S106.

Viens, A. M. (2019). Neo-liberalism, austerity and the political determinants of health, *Health Care Analysis*, 27, 147–152.

Waitzkin, H. (2020). Moving beyond capitalism for our health. *International Journal of Health Services*, 50(4), 458–462.

Weil, A. (2020). Tackling social determinants of health around the globe, *Health Affairs*, 39(7), 118–1121.

West, R. & Marteau, T. (2013). Commentary on Casswell: the commercial determinants of health, *Addiction*, 108(4), 686–687.

World Health Organization. (1948). Constitution. Retrieved from www.who.int/about/governance/constitution.

Yamin, A. E. (2019). Struggles for human rights in health in an age of neoliberalism: From civil disobedience to epistemic disobedience, *Journal of Human Rights Practice*, 11(2), 357–372.

Yuill, C., Crinson, I. & Duncan, E. (2010). *Key Concepts in Health Studies*, Thousand Oaks, CA: Sage Publications.

Zola, I. (1977). Healthism and disabling medicalization. In I. Illich (ed.), *Disabling Professions*, London: Marion Boyars.

4 Compassion in Healthcare

Debbie Ling

Introduction

Compassion is a core value in health care and fundamental to social work practice. Social workers hold that every human being has a unique and inherent equal worth (Australian Association of Social Workers 2020). The social work profession is founded on the principles of the United Nations Universal Declaration of Human Rights (United Nations 1948). Social workers strive to maximise the physical, mental and social wellbeing of individuals and society. Social work practice in health care can involve complex situations where social workers may need to make difficult decisions. Compassion, with its focus on alleviating the suffering of the other, provides the basis upon which social workers can choose the most constructive course of action to take.

Compassion is now understood to have an evolutionary benefit: it is essential for caregivers to recognise and respond when their offspring are unwell or in need. Caring and connection to others is the foundation of functioning societies. Recent research has revealed that compassion also has clear benefits for the giver, not just the recipient, of compassion. Compassion promotes the wellbeing of the giver and is protective against burnout. Social workers in health care are regularly working with people who may be distressed and the social worker needs to have a compassionate response to be able to fulfil their role. There is now significant interest in how to train and strengthen compassion.

What Is Compassion?

Although compassion has been acknowledged as a virtue across cultures for centuries, it has only recently become a topic of research interest. Compassion research is in its infancy and is not yet prominent in social work literature or curricula (Tanner 2020). Compassion is defined as 'the feeling that arises in witnessing another's suffering and that motivates a subsequent desire to help' (Goetz et al. 2010: 352).

Compassion leads to benefits for patients' physical health (DiMatteo et al. 1993; Graser et al. 2018), improves the psychological health of the patient (Fogarty et al. 1999; Kemper et al. 2011; Kok et al. 2013; Shaltout et al. 2012); improves the quality of care (Patel et al. 2019) and improves the wellbeing of the health care worker (Fredrickson et al. 2008; Klimecki et al. 2013). Compassion has been shown to reduce stress in the caregiver (Dahl et al. 2015), reduce depression in the caregiver (Mascaro et al. 2018) and reduce the desire to punish the other (Condon & DeSteno 2011). Compassion has a positive impact on those who witness it (Kanov et al. 2004). Neuroscience research has even demonstrated that compassion is a positive state of mind and leads to feelings of

DOI: 10.4324/9781003330745-5

warmth, concern, reward and affiliation (Klimecki et al. 2013, Preckel et al. 2018). There is now a recognition that humans are social animals and that prosocial behaviours such as caring, connection and compassion are a fundamental part of being human (Dunbar 1998). There is evidence that helping others, 'helper's high', boosts the wellbeing of the giver (Post 2011).

Compassion and Empathy are Not the Same

Despite the acknowledged centrality of compassion in health care, there is some confusion regarding understanding compassion (Kirby 2017; Strauss et al. 2016). Social workers have been found to have different interpretations in relation to what they understand compassion to be (Ortega-Galán et al. 2020).

Compassion is often used interchangeably with other terms such as pity, empathy and sympathy which can lead to confusion. Pity is where one may feel sorry for someone else but it involves an aspect of looking down upon the other (Von Dietze & Orb 2000). Empathy is where we are affected by and share another's feelings (Gilbert 2010). Sympathy is where we feel sorry for another but lack the extra step of wishing to alleviate their suffering (Ricard 2015). It is most important to make the distinction between compassion and empathy. Compassion and empathy have distinct neural pathways (Klimecki et al. 2013). Empathy has two aspects, cognitive and affective (see Figure 4.1).

Cognitive empathy is where one can take the perspective of another and understand their situation. Affective empathy is where one feels with the other and has an emotional resonance with them. When confronted with another's suffering, empathy may accidentally turn into empathic distress, which is where the social worker becomes overwhelmed by their own personal distress. This may be due to imagining the other's pain or can be a self-focused thought such as 'I can't deal with this today' or 'I have a meeting to go to in five minutes and don't have time for this'. Social workers may also wish to avoid others who are suffering if the social worker finds themselves going into personal distress too often (see Figure 4.2).

It is important to understand that empathy is a *feeling* state: it does not necessarily lead to action. Compassion goes beyond empathy (Ortega-Galán et al. 2020). Compassion is a wish to alleviate the suffering of another, which is the motivation for caring *actions*.

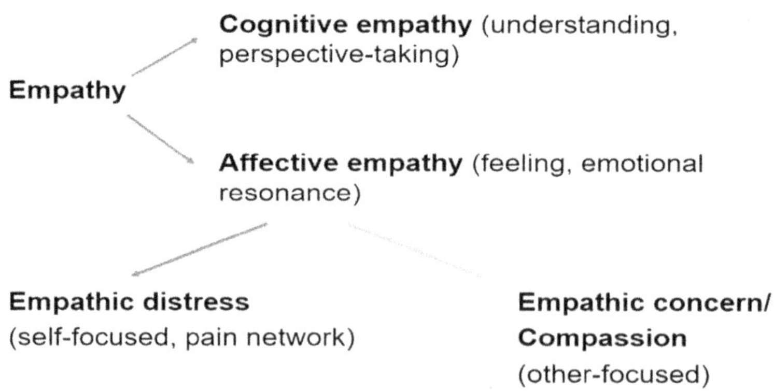

Figure 4.1 Cognitive empathy and affective empathy

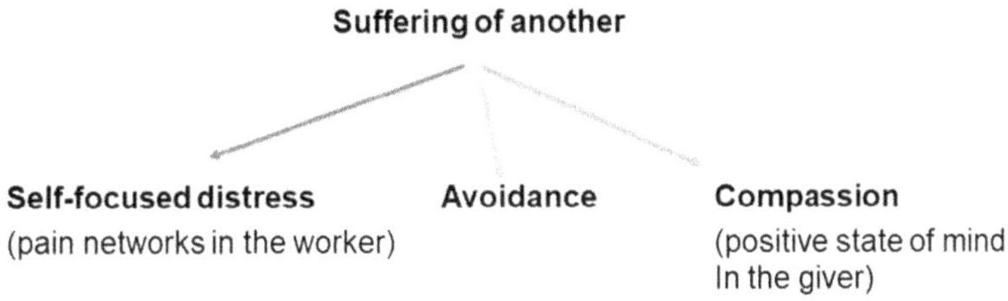

Figure 4.2 Responses to the suffering of another

Compassion is not a simple emotion but is a complex response involving:

Perception → Empathy → Motivation to relieve the suffering of the other

There are several points in this response where compassion may not arise. First, the social worker needs to be aware that the other is suffering. Sometimes a social worker will not be able to tune into the other if the social worker has a high caseload and multiple demands. Being in a hurry and self-absorbed has been shown to inhibit helping behaviour (Darley & Batson 1973). Second, the social worker needs to keep their empathy response focused on the other and not have it accidentally turn into self-focused personal distress, now called empathic distress. Third, the social worker is required to make a connection with the other and wish for the suffering of the other to be relieved. A situation where this may not occur is if the social worker considers the other person is not deserving of compassion. It is known that healthcare workers can make moral judgements about patients (Hill 2010).

It is important to acknowledge that not all suffering can be prevented. Social workers often work with people who may have complex or chronic health condition where 'fixing' the health issue may not be possible at that time. Some social workers may inhibit a compassionate response if they consider they cannot alleviate the suffering of the other. Nevertheless, in these circumstances, a compassionate response from the social worker is still the most valuable response, both for themselves and the person they are working with.

Compassion as an Antidote to Empathic Distress

Social workers in health care may be confronted multiple times per day with others who are suffering. Social work can be a stressful occupation (Senreich et al. 2020). It is important for social workers to have a clear understanding of the difference between compassion and empathic distress (self-focused personal distress). If a social worker is unwittingly responding to another's suffering with empathic distress, it is possible this will lead to burn out for the worker. Equally, a social worker may start to wish to avoid the suffering of the other as a self-protective response. Whilst this is understandable as a short-term strategy, it does not benefit the social worker or the patient. The term 'compassion fatigue' which has been popular for the last two decades is now understood to be incorrectly named: it is actually 'empathic distress fatigue' (Hofmeyer et al. 2020). Compassion and empathy have distinct neural pathways (Ashar et al. 2017; Klimecki & Singer 2012). Compassion is a positive neural pathway and leads to wellbeing benefits in the social worker. However if the social worker is accidentally remaining in an emotional resonance with their patients' distress and/or becoming distressed themselves, then there is a risk of burnout.

Working in health care places many demands on all members of the multidisciplinary team. There can be high workloads, systems pressures, resource issues and differences of opinion. Compassion is critical not just in the worker-to-patient relationship but also in the worker-to-worker relationship. However, compassion is rarely the focus of training programs (Stickle 2016). Social work educators will play a key role in preparing future graduates with the appropriate skills for working in complex environments (Udah & Francis 2021). There is increased interest in compassionate leadership and how to foster compassionate workplaces. Social workers are well placed to support such initiatives, given the social work understanding of person-in-environment and systems theory. It is important for organisations to have adequate supervision, peer support and peer debriefing programs. The COVID pandemic has highlighted the intense pressure on the healthcare sector with high demand on health care, mental health, family violence, unemployment and crisis services.

Common Humanity as the Prerequisite for Unbiased Universal Compassion

People may have compassion for their close others or those they consider similar to themselves. However people do not always have compassion for those they consider less deserving of compassion or for out-group members. According to the values of social work, it is important to respect the inherent dignity and worth of every person (Australian Association of Social Workers 2020). Social work practice is based on an understanding of 'person-in-environment', that is, there are a range of factors that influence people's choices and behaviour at any point in time. Social determinants of health, for example, poverty, unemployment, education, social exclusion etc. play a key role in people's health and access to services. Social work has a commitment to working with anyone in need, for example social workers can be found working with those who have committed crimes as well as those who have been the victims of crime. Respect for human dignity means that irrespective of any past action in their lives, the fundamental humanity of the person must be valued. There are instances where people may have intersected with the criminal justice system at a point in their lives and have subsequently undergone rehabilitation and gone on to contribute to society in meaningful ways.

Compassion in health care requires social workers to have a compassionate response to every person they work with, and not make a judgement on whether or not the person deserves compassion. This is not always easy to do. Social workers, like anyone else, can have biases and prejudices they are unaware of. It is known that people tend to favour in-group members (Amodio 2008; Tajfel 1982), but also that group membership can change, depending on context (Turner et al. 1994). The ability to view others from the perspective of a shared humanity brings everyone into the in-group. This enables the social worker to make a connection with any other person.

The perception of common humanity has been proposed to be the prerequisite for unbiased universal compassion (Blum 1980; Cassell 2009; Jinpa 2016; Ling et al. 2020; Monroe 1998; Von Dietze & Orb 2000). Common humanity involves understanding that (i) all people share the same wish to be happy and not to suffer, (ii) the universality of suffering as part of the human condition and (iii) having a sense of gratitude and appreciation of others due to understanding the interconnected nature of human relationships. Every human has been the recipient of another's compassion, even if it was at the beginning of their lives as a baby where it took many years of caregiver resources and attention to raise them. People especially appreciate the care and kindness of others when they are at their most vulnerable, which is often the case if they are unwell and needing to access health care services.

Reviewing all the people who may have ever helped, supported or positively influenced oneself, even if in a fleeting way, can heighten one's sense of the importance of other people's acts of kindness. Societies with a strong individualised focus tend not to consciously reflect how there is no 'self-made person'. Any single individual has necessarily been the recipient of help, support and resources from multiple others, including the level of education. Reviewing their own experience of common humanity can help social workers understand the impact of their actions on others in their daily work.

How Does a Patient Experience Compassion?

It is common for health care organisations to have compassion as a stated core value. Patients and service users expect to be treated with compassion (Frampton et al. 2013; Lown et al. 2011; Sharp et al. 2016). Bramley and Matiti (2014) report that patients said they experienced compassion when they felt the health care worker related to them as a person, gave them time and communicated in a compassionate manner. In addition, Sinclair et al. (2016) found that patients reported they experienced compassion when the worker listened to them, attended to their needs, sought to understand them without judgment and engaged in helping behaviours. The key ingredients that comprise a compassionate response appear to be attending, empathy, understanding, no judgement and kindness. These qualities can manifest in a range of ways including verbal interactions, responding to physical care needs, emotional support, following up on requests for information, involving family and carers, communication with the wider team and advocating for other support services.

Blocks to Compassion

There are multiple issues, both internal and external to the social worker that can block the arising of compassion.

Internal issues can include:

- being distracted and not able place their attention upon the other;
- being unaware the other is suffering;
- empathic distress;
- a judgment that the other is not deserving of compassion;
- believing one does not have a solution for the situation; and
- believing that compassion is 'too soft'.

External issues can include:

- excessive workloads;
- negative work culture;
- systems which dehumanise the patient; and
- team conflict.

It is useful if the social worker can strengthen their own awareness of the types of issues that may be impacting on their compassionate response to others. Once aware of the issues, the social worker is better placed to take action to address the issues. This may involve working on their own core beliefs and emotional regulation or advocating for fairer workloads and culture change.

Reflection: Dan's Story

Dan is a 23-year-old man from regional Victoria. He was living in Office of Housing accommodation and was on JobSeeker benefits payment. Dan was a regular user and dealer of heroin and was also growing marijuana in a homemade drug lab to sell for profit. There was an accident in Dan's drug lab and he sustained serious burns to 60% of his body, most severely in his lower body. Dan has four step-brothers and step-sisters, but he is not close to them. He has intermittent contact with his mother with whom he is also not close. Whilst Dan was semi-conscious in intensive care, one of his step-brothers visited him and managed to get Dan's PIN number for his bank account and he removed $3,000 that Dan had in the account. Dan was upset when he discovered this but was unable to get back in touch with his step-brother or recover his money.

Dan required multiple operations to address his serious burns and he was in an inpatient rehabilitation ward for 9 months. Due to the severity of his burns, Dan is now in a wheelchair and unlikely to walk again however Dan cannot accept this and still hopes to recover his ability to walk. The public hospital ward has strict rules about not using drugs whilst in hospital. Unfortunately Dan broke this rule and was discovered to have started using heroin that he had obtained from a friend. Dan was also having some drug dealer friends visit him on the ward. The multidisciplinary team had a meeting with Dan, explained the rules around no drug use and cautioned Dan to stop using or he would be discharged from hospital. Dan was made to undergo compulsory drug tests. Dan failed his drug tests two days in a row and the consulting doctor made the decision to discharge Dan immediately from the ward, despite his rehabilitation being incomplete. Dan had nowhere to go as his housing had also been destroyed in the fire.

Reflection Questions

1 You are the social worker on the ward. Do you think the decision to discharge Dan immediately is a compassionate response?
2 Given Dan is in a wheelchair and has no appropriate accommodation to go to, what do you think are the options?
3 The multidisciplinary team is not always in agreement regarding patient care. What do you see as the role of the social worker in Dan's situation?

What Constitutes a Compassionate Social Work Response?

Compassion provides the motivation to take action to alleviate the suffering of another. There is no one specific answer regarding how compassion is translated into action. Each person's health situation is specific to them. The social worker has to consider each individual circumstance before deciding upon a course of action. Social workers may undertake a range of actions in pursuit of enhancing the wellbeing of others. Advocating for the rights of those who may not be in a position to speak up for themselves is a core part of social work practice. A compassionate response may also be a firm response. For example, a social worker may be needed to advocate to the multidisciplinary team or other service providers for more services on behalf of someone with complex health issues. Or a social worker may need to take a mediating role if there is disagreement within a family regarding how to best support someone. Occasionally a social worker may need to take stronger steps such as making a referral to child protection or mental health services if they believe the safety of someone is at risk. A compassionate response is about the social worker determining the most constructive course of action that will maximise the health and wellbeing of the other.

Reflection: Working in Multidisciplinary Teams

Social workers in health care often work in multidisciplinary teams. Whilst health professionals all have the same aim – a genuine desire to improve the health outcome of the patient – teams do not always agree on the plan regarding how to achieve this. The social work role requires the workers to consult closely with the patient and family and then advocate for the best interests of the patient and family. At times, this can require expressing an opinion which is counter to what the team wishes to do. It is not always easy to be the dissenting opinion.

Reflection Questions

1. Compassion means placing the patient's interests first and foremost. How might this be challenging for you as the social worker on the team?
2. Disagreement is a fact of life at times. Have you ever been in a situation where you had to disagree with a work colleague and, if so, how did you handle it?
3. Learning to work through complex situations which require difficult decisions is a normal part of life as a social worker. What are some phrases which might be helpful to use?

Creating Compassionate Workplaces

Compassion in the workplace is increasingly considered as an essential component of workplaces that function well (Dutton et al. 2014; Lilius et al. 2008). Those who are compassionate create supportive interpersonal environments for themselves and others (Crocker & Canevello 2008). There is an increasing focus on the need for compassionate leadership (de Zulueta 2016). Social workers can play a major role in helping facilitate positive work environments as social workers are trained to support discussion on difficult topics. Often the busy nature of work in health care settings means there is a lack of opportunities for teams to debrief and to reflect on ensuring they are providing the best services for the service users. Teams themselves also need to track their own wellbeing.

It is acknowledged that compassion has, at times, been lacking in health care (Francis 2013; Youngson 2011). Social work advocacy may play an important role in assisting organisations to embed compassion in the workplace. Social workers and other health care workers are at risk of burnout due to the demanding nature of their work. Health care organisations have a primary responsibility to provide compassionate care to the service users. It is imperative that there are efforts made to support the creation of compassionate workplaces. To truly embed compassion in the workplace, bottom-up approaches, such as providing compassion training to staff, are an important option but have their limitations. There also needs to be top-down initiatives, where management and leadership not only act as role models of compassionate behaviours but assist in the creation of a compassionate workplace culture.

Conclusion

Compassion is considered the foundation of health care. Service users and patients expect to receive compassionate care. Compassion is also the central foundation underpinning social work values and principles. Research is revealing an increased understanding of the distinction between compassion and other related terms, in particular, empathy. When confronted by the suffering of others, the social worker's ability to keep their focus on compassion appears to be an important strategy to avoid empathic distress and burnout. The perception of common humanity helps social workers maintain a prosocial perspective towards every person with whom they work. Social workers are skilled at employing a range of compassionate approaches in their work in health. Social workers are a core part of health service delivery and will probably play important roles in the future in helping embed compassion in health settings.

Key Website Resources

United Nations (www.un.org/en).

Charter for Compassion Australia (www.charterforcompassion.com.au).

References

Amodio, D. M. (2008). The social neuroscience of intergroup relations. *European Review of Social Psychology*, 19(1), 1–54.

Ashar, Y. K., Andrews-Hanna, J. R., Dimidjian, S. & Wager, T. D. (2017). Empathic care and distress: predictive brain markers and dissociable brain systems. *Neuron*, 94(6), 1263–1273.

Australian Association of Social Workers. (2020). *Code of ethics*. Canberra: AASW.

Blum, L. (1980). *Compassion*. In A. O. Rorty (ed.), *Explaining emotions*, 507–571. Berkeley, CA: University of California Press.

Bramley, L. & Matiti, M. (2014). How does it really feel to be in my shoes? Patients' experiences of compassion within nursing care and their perceptions of developing compassionate nurses. *Journal of Clinical Nursing*, 23(19–20), 2790–2799.

Cassell, E. J. (2009). Compassion. In C. R. Snyder & S. J. Lopez (eds), *Oxford handbook of positive psychology*, 393–404. Oxford: Oxford University Press.

Condon, P. & DeSteno, D. (2011). Compassion for one reduces punishment for another. *Journal of Experimental Social Psychology*, 47(3), 698–701.

Crocker, J. & Canevello, A. (2008). 'Creating and undermining social support in communal relationships: the role of compassionate and self-image goals'. *Journal of Personality and Social Psychology*, 95(3), 555.

Dahl, C. J., Lutz, A. & Davidson, R. J. (2015). Reconstructing and deconstructing the self: cognitive mechanisms in meditation practice. *Trends in Cognitive Sciences*, 19(9), 515–523.

Darley, J. M. & Batson, C. D. (1973). 'From Jerusalem to Jericho': A study of situational and dispositional variables in helping behavior. *Journal of Personality and Social Psychology*, 27(1), 100.

de Zulueta, P. C. (2016). Developing compassionate leadership in health care: an integrative review. *Journal of Healthcare Leadership*, 8, 1.

DiMatteo, M. R., Sherbourne, C. D., Hays, R. D., Ordway, L., Kravitz, R. L., McGlynn, E. A., Kaplan, S. & Rogers, W. H. (1993). Physicians' characteristics influence patients' adherence to medical treatment: results from the Medical Outcomes Study. *Health Psychology*, 12(2), 93.

Dunbar, R. I. (1998). The social brain hypothesis. *Evolutionary Anthropology: Issues, News, and Reviews: Issues, News, and Reviews*, 6(5), 178–190.

Durkin, J., Usher, K. & Jackson, D. (2019). Embodying compassion: A systematic review of the views of nurses and patients. *Journal of Clinical Nursing*, 28(9–10), 1380–1392.

Dutton, J. E., Workman, K. M. & Hardin, A. E. (2014). Compassion at work. *Annual Review of Organizational Psychology and Organizational Behavior*, 1(1), 277–304.

Fogarty, L. A., Curbow, B. A., Wingard, J. R., McDonnell, K. & Somerfield, M. R. (1999). Can 40 seconds of compassion reduce patient anxiety? *Journal of Clinical Oncology*, 17(1), pp.371–371.

Frampton, S. B., Guastello, S. & Lepore, M. (2013). Compassion as the foundation of patient-centered care: the importance of compassion in action. *Journal of Comparative Effectiveness Research*, 2(5), 443–455.

Francis, R. (2013). *Report of the Mid Staffordshire NHS Foundation Trust public inquiry: executive summary* (vol. 947). The Stationery Office.

Fredrickson, B. L., Cohn, M. A., Coffey, K. A., Pek, J. & Finkel, S. M. (2008). Open hearts build lives: positive emotions, induced through loving-kindness meditation, build consequential personal resources. *Journal of Personality and Social Psychology*, 95(5), 1045.

Gilbert, P. (2010). *The compassionate mind: A new approach to life's challenges*. New Harbinger Publications.

Goetz, J. L., Keltner, D. & Simon-Thomas, E. (2010). Compassion: an evolutionary analysis and empirical review. *Psychological Bulletin*, 136(3), 351.

Graser, J. & Stangier, U. (2018). Compassion and loving-kindness meditation: an overview and prospects for the application in clinical samples. *Harvard Review of Psychiatry*, 26(4), 201–215.

Hill, T. E. (2010). How clinicians make (or avoid) moral judgments of patients: implications of the evidence for relationships and research. *Philosophy, Ethics, and Humanities in Medicine*, 5(1), 1–14.

Hofmeyer, A., Kennedy, K. & Taylor, R. (2020). Contesting the term 'compassion fatigue': Integrating findings from social neuroscience and self-care research. *Collegian*, 27(2), 232–237.

Iyengar, S., Lelkes, Y., Levendusky, M., Malhotra, N. & Westwood, S. J. (2019). The origins and consequences of affective polarization in the United States. *Annual Review of Political Science*, 22, 129–146.

Jinpa, T. (2016). *A fearless heart: How the courage to be compassionate can transform our lives*. Avery.

Kanov, J. M., Maitlis, S., Worline, M. C., Dutton, J. E., Frost, P. J. & Lilius, J. M. (2004). Compassion in organizational life. *American Behavioral Scientist*, 47(6), 808–827.

Kemper, K. J. & Shaltout, H.A. (2011). Non-verbal communication of compassion: measuring psychophysiologic effects. *BMC Complementary and Alternative Medicine*, 11(1), 1–9.

Kirby, J. N. (2017). Compassion interventions: The programmes, the evidence, and implications for research and practice. *Psychology and Psychotherapy: Theory, Research and Practice*, 90(3), 432–455.

Klimecki, O. & Singer, T. (2012). Empathic distress fatigue rather than compassion fatigue? Integrating findings from empathy research in psychology and social neuroscience. In B. Oakley, A. Knafo, G. Madhavan & D. S. Wilson (eds), *Pathological altruism*, 368–383. Oxford: Oxford University Press.

Klimecki, O. M., Leiberg, S., Ricard, M. & Singer, T. (2013). Differential pattern of functional brain plasticity after compassion and empathy training. *Social cognitive and affective neuroscience*, 9(6), 873–879.

Kok, B. E., Coffey, K. A., Cohn, M. A., Catalino, L. I., Vacharkulksemsuk, T., Algoe, S. B., Brantley, M. & Fredrickson, B. L. (2013). How positive emotions build physical health: Perceived positive social connections account for the upward spiral between positive emotions and vagal tone. *Psychological science*, 24(7), 1123–1132.

Lilius, J. M., Worline, M. C., Maitlis, S., Kanov, J., Dutton, J. E. & Frost, P. (2008). The contours and consequences of compassion at work. *Journal of Organizational Behavior*, 29(2), 193–218.

Ling, D., Olver, J. & Petrakis, M. (2020). Investigating how viewing common humanity scenarios impacts compassion: a novel approach. *The British Journal of Social Work*, 50(6), 1724–1742.

Lown, B. A., Rosen, J. & Marttila, J. (2011). An agenda for improving compassionate care: a survey shows about half of patients say such care is missing. *Health Affairs*, 30(9), 1772–1778.

Mascaro, J. S., Kelley, S., Darcher, A., Negi, L. T., Worthman, C., Miller, A. & Raison, C. (2018). Meditation buffers medical student compassion from the deleterious effects of depression. *The Journal of Positive Psychology*, 13(2), 133–142.

Monroe, K. R. (1998). *The heart of altruism: Perceptions of a common humanity*. Princeton, NJ: Princeton University Press.

Ortega-Galán, Á. M., Ruiz-Fernández, M. D. & Ortíz-Amo, R. (2020). Compassion and empathy in community social workers: A qualitative study in Spain. *Health & Social Care in the Community*, 29(5), 1349–1358.

Patel, S., Pelletier-Bui, A., Smith, S., Roberts, M. B., Kilgannon, H., Trzeciak, S. & Roberts, B. W. (2019). Curricula for empathy and compassion training in medical education: a systematic review. *PLoS One*, 14(8), e0221412.

Post, S. G. (2011). It's good to be good: 2011 fifth annual scientific report on health, happiness and helping others. *International Journal of Person Centered Medicine*, 1(4), 814–829.

Preckel, K., Kanske, P. & Singer, T. (2018). On the interaction of social affect and cognition: empathy, compassion and theory of mind. *Current Opinion in Behavioral Sciences*, 19, 1–6.

Ricard, M. (2015). *Altruism: The power of compassion to change yourself and the world*. New York: Atlantic Books.

Senreich, E., Straussner, S. L. A. & Steen, J. (2020). The work experiences of social workers: Factors impacting compassion satisfaction and workplace stress. *Journal of Social Service Research*, 46(1), 93–109.

Sharp, S., McAllister, M. & Broadbent, M. (2016). The vital blend of clinical competence and compassion: How patients experience person-centred care. *Contemporary Nurse*, 52(2–3), 300–312.

Shaltout, H. A., Tooze, J. A., Rosenberger, E. & Kemper, K. J. (2012). Time, touch, and compassion: Effects on autonomic nervous system and well-being. *Explore*, 8(3), 177–184.

Sinclair, S., McClement, S., Raffin-Bouchal, S., Hack, T. F., Hagen, N. A., McConnell, S. & Chochinov, H. M. (2016). Compassion in health care: an empirical model. *Journal of Pain and Symptom Management*, 51(2), 193–203.

Stickle, M. (2016). The expression of compassion in social work practice. *Journal of Religion & Spirituality in Social Work: Social Thought*, 35(1–2), 120–131.

Strauss, C., Taylor, B. L., Gu, J., Kuyken, W., Baer, R., Jones, F. & Cavanagh, K. (2016). What is compassion and how can we measure it? A review of definitions and measures. *Clinical Psychology Review*, 47, 15–27.

Tajfel, H. (1982). Social psychology of intergroup relations. *Annual Review of Psychology*, 33(1), 1–39.

Tanner, D. (2020). 'The love that dare not speak its name': The role of compassion in social work practice. *The British Journal of Social Work*, 50(6), 1688–1705.

Trowbridge, K. & Mische Lawson, L. (2016). Mindfulness-based interventions with social workers and the potential for enhanced patient-centered care: A systematic review of the literature. *Social Work in Health Care*, 55(2), 101–124.

Turner, J. C., Oakes, P. J., Haslam, S. A. & McGarty, C. (1994). Self and collective: Cognition and social context. *Personality and Social Psychology Bulletin*, 20(5), 454–463.

Udah, H. & Francis, A. (2021). COVID-19: Challenges, opportunities, and the future of social work. *International Journal of Innovation, Creativity and Change*, 15, 54–74.

United Nations. (1948). The universal declaration of human rights. Retrieved from www.un.org/en/about-us/universal-declaration-of-human-rights.

Vaillant, G. E. (2008). *Aging well: Surprising guideposts to a happier life from the landmark study of adult development*. London: Hachette UK.

Von Dietze, E. & Orb, A. (2000). Compassionate care: a moral dimension of nursing. *Nursing Inquiry*, 7(3), 166–174.

Wagner, M. (2021). Affective polarization in multiparty systems. *Electoral Studies*, 69, 102199.

Youngson, R. (2011). Compassion in healthcare – the missing dimension of healthcare reform. In I. Renzenbrink (ed.), *Caregiver stress and staff support in illness, dying, and bereavement*, 49–61. Oxford: Oxford University Press.

Part II

Health Practice and Practice Contexts

5 Trauma-Informed Practices in Health Social Work

Margaret Cowgill and Rose Knol

Introduction

The role of a social worker in an acute hospital trauma setting can be emotionally intense and complex. It is a fast-paced environment and there is a need to be prepared for any situation. There can be wide-ranging and far-reaching psychosocial implications for the injured person. In circumstances of major trauma admissions, the social worker meets with people when their world has suddenly been turned upside down. Traumatic events can bring people together; however, traumatic events can also exacerbate pre-existing social issues and place relationships under enormous strain. In this context the social worker's role is to understand the biomedical aspects and assess the psychosocial factors at play, while working to contain the crisis, address issues and provide resources. This will be done amid all the demands of working in a hospital system.

Occasionally people may be admitted to hospital with injuries sustained due to either natural disasters (for example, bushfires and earthquakes) or man-made incidents that result in mass casualties and require coordinated specialist support; in these instances the psychological trauma can extend to whole communities.

Despite its challenges, working in the area of hospital trauma can also be very rewarding because the social worker is required to utilise the various dimensions of knowledge and theory of social work practice. This chapter is designed to provide an outline of the role of a hospital social worker in a trauma ward, from specific single-issue interventions to the more complex work required. It includes an overview of the type of acute trauma reactions workers may be required to attempt to alleviate, and the support available to social workers. The latter is very important for career longevity and self-care.

What Is Trauma?

Trauma is a significant health problem and cause of death worldwide. In Australia between 2017 and 2018, traumatic injuries accounted for the long-term health conditions of more than 300,000 people living with a disability (AIHW, 2020). Physical trauma is an injury to the body caused by an external force and in Australia the leading causes of traumatic injury are falls, road traffic accidents, being struck by an object or person, self-harm, burns and horse-related injuries. Worldwide, older adults are more likely to be admitted due to falls and younger adults are more likely to be admitted with self-inflicted traumatic injuries, often with pre-existing mental health issues (Devassy & Varghese, 2020; Veselsky et al., 2021). Psychologically, McCann and Pearlman (1990) define trauma as: '(1) sudden, unexpected or non-normative, (2), exceeds the person's perceived ability

DOI: 10.4324/9781003330745-7

to meet its demands, and (3) disrupts the individual's frame of reference and other central psychological needs and related schema's'.

A patient being overseen by a trauma team will generally have more than one injury, and be receiving surgical support from more than one group of doctors; for example orthopaedic surgeons will be managing the fractures, neuro-surgeons will be treating a head injury, burns injuries will be managed by burns and plastics specialists, and a pre-existing or trauma-caused illness will be monitored by medical doctors. In some cases a psychiatric team may also be assessing and treating a patient.

Impact of COVID-19 on Trauma and Admissions

In Australia and in many other countries, lockdowns have meant that large proportions of the population have been restricted to their homes and have had to adhere to strict social distancing rules. This has directly impacted on the type and frequency of trauma admissions world-wide, for example, studies have shown a significant decrease in trauma admissions related to traffic collisions (Kamine et al., 2020; Jacob et al., 2020; Harris et al., 2021). Similarly, a comparison of facial injury presentations across tertiary hospitals in Australia and the UK found a noticeable decrease in interpersonal violence as the cause (Hoffman et al., 2020).

Research has identified that restrictions imposed to better control the pandemic have also had negative unforeseen consequences, for example injuries relating to family violence have increased since the pandemic started (Waseem et al., 2020; Hoffman et al., 2020; Olding et al., 2021; Van Gelder et al., 2020). Social isolation and reduced work and income, have increased risk factors of intimate partner and family violence (Olding et al., 2021; Van Gelder et al., 2020) and studies have shown an increase in penetrating and burn injuries related to self-harm during 2020–2021 (Olding et al., 2021; Marques et al., 2021). Not unexpectedly a further area of increased trauma has been injuries in and around the house such as falls (Harris et al., 2021; Waseem et al., 2020) and burns.

Another consequence of the pandemic on health care has been restricting visitors to prevent and/or manage outbreaks of infection in hospitals. While the reasoning behind these policies is clear, the consequences have been detrimental to patients and their significant others. The benefits of patient and family involvement in their health care and the importance of informal social support in physical and psychological recovery are well known (Silvera et al., 2021). Not having this type of support has been shown to increase the safety risks of patients in areas such as falls and reduced nutrition; as well as being a cause of psychological distress and loneliness (Munshi et al., 2021; Silvera et al., 2021). It has also increased the level of carer anxiety, and their need for information and social support (Hugelius et al., 2021).

Social workers have provided creative interventions to support patients and their families 'meeting' together and having regular updates from the patient's treating team. Understanding the impact of the pandemic and how factors such as social isolation and quarantine can affect trauma presentations, risk, and available interventions, is crucial when conducting a psychosocial assessment.

Acute Traumatic Stress

Traumatic stress can impact not only the person injured, but also those who witnessed the event, those who learn of a close family member or friend being impacted, and those who experience repeated exposure to details of the event (for example, emergency and support workers). According to Hopper et al. (2010), 'Trauma refers to an experience that creates a sense of fear, helplessness or horror and overwhelms a person's resources for coping. It potentially poses a threat to one's life, safety or personal integrity.'

Trauma reaches well beyond the physical impact of the injury. In terms of psychosocial responses to traumatic injury, Tedeschi and Calhoun (1995) state four key characteristics of traumatic events: they are 'sudden and unexpected', 'out of one's control' and 'out of the ordinary', and they 'create long lasting problems'.

The Diagnostic and Statistical Manual (DSM) is used by psychiatrists to diagnose mental health disorders and may guide other care professionals. The most recent version, the DSM V, lists five types of acute stress reactions:

1 Intrusion symptoms: include recurrent, involuntary and intrusive distressing memories; flashbacks and intense or prolonged psychological distress;
2 Negative mood: an inability to experience positive emotions; for example, happiness, satisfaction or loving feelings with regard to self and others;
3 Dissociative symptoms: an altered sense of reality, that may include seeing oneself from another's perspective, being in a daze, time slowing, not remembering important aspects of the traumatic events (dissociative amnesia);
4 Avoidance symptoms: avoiding distressing memories, thoughts or feelings related to the traumatic event; avoiding external reminders – people, places, conversations, activities, objects, situations – that may arouse distressing memories, thoughts, or feelings;
5 Arousal symptoms: disturbed sleep, irritability and anger; verbal and physical aggression to others or objects; hypervigilance, yet also an inability to concentrate, and being easily startled.

Social workers are often called upon to assist someone to manage symptoms of traumatic stress. When symptoms persist, seeking formal support is encouraged. Strategies that might be useful to use with clients in psychoeducation, and as mental health first aid, are covered in detail at the website 'Better Health Channel: Trauma – Reaction and Recovery' (see web link at the end of this chapter). Some common approaches are summarised below.

Biopsychosocial Dimensions of Traumatic Injury

It cannot be predicted how a person will respond to trauma nor their risk of developing long-term mental health issues. The biopsychosocial assessment (Figure 5.1) is an essential tool to enable the social worker to identify risk factors and understand the psychological and/or social factors that may impact on a person's reaction, treatment and recovery. As noted by Sayed et al. (2015): 'Risk factors for the development of psychopathology following trauma exposure fall into three categories: pre-trauma, peri-trauma and post-trauma factors. Pre-trauma factors can include age, gender, race/ethnicity, education, prior psychopathology, and neurobiological factors. Peri-trauma factors can include the duration/severity of trauma experience and the perception that the trauma has ended. Post-trauma factors can include access to needed resources, social support, specific cognitive patterns, and physical activity.'

Emotional reactions to a traumatic incident are expected and vary from person to person; they generally subside over time, however, when people have ongoing distressing reactions, support should be encouraged.

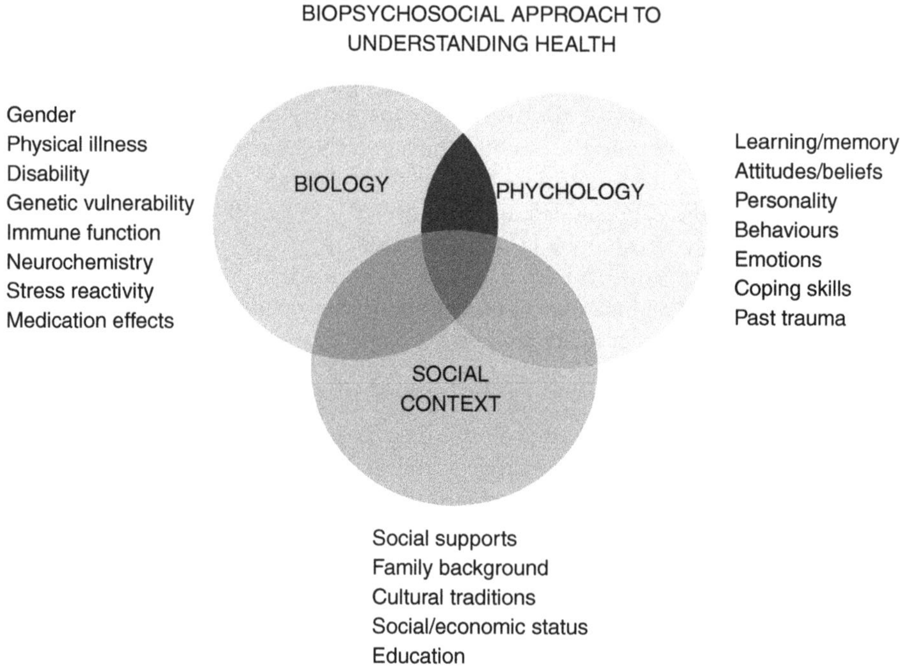

Figure 5.1 The biopsychosocial model of health
Source: http://perspectivesclinic.com/health-psychology

Reflection: Jane's Story

Tim, an acute trauma social worker, was referred to see Jane as she had been experiencing distressing flashbacks of her motor vehicle accident. Jane was the single occupant in her car when she went around a corner and the car flipped over several times. Jane has neck and spinal injuries and so was lying flat on her back in a body and neck brace.

Tim began the session by sitting so that Jane could see him comfortably, and asking Jane questions about herself, her family, job, any practical concerns she may be having. This provided context and information about Jane's supports and her life outside of the hospital, as well as developing rapport. Overall, Jane spoke of having a positive and fulfilling life in that she has a successful job, supportive parents, and is planning on getting married in the next year.

Tim then led Jane into discussion about the accident by firstly asking if she wanted to talk about it. In this instance Jane did, however patients can find the talking process too traumatising and in those situations their preference should be respected. Jane described the accident calmly and without noticeable distress, however she became more agitated when talking about being upside down and unable to take off her seatbelt. This is the event Jane has been seeing over again in flashbacks and waking nightmares. Tim was able to explore Jane's feelings gently and supportively until she could articulate that her greatest fear had been another car coming and hitting her while she was still trapped. This possible scenario had caused Jane to feel very unsafe and very vulnerable.

Tim was able to acknowledge and reassure Jane that these fears are understandable, and went on to provide psychoeducation regarding trauma responses, and how our minds can continue to go over events as a means of understanding and processing them. Tim also suggested that Jane may continue to feel vulnerable and unsafe given she is in an unfamiliar environment with injuries that are preventing her from moving. Jane understood that her usual way of dealing with stress (going to the gym, bike riding) was not possible. Tim was able to introduce ways of managing the flashbacks when they occurred, by teaching Jane grounding techniques to bring her back to the here and now, and suggesting she practise mindfulness, or use mindfulness apps that she can access on her phone.

Reflection Questions

1 What key theory or theories are informing Tim's approach with this patient?
2 How is Tim using the biopsychosocial model of health to inform his assessment?
3 Tim is having to manage competing demands – at what point should he end involvement with Jane?

Specific Interventions That Social Workers Apply in the Acute Setting

Crisis Support/Psychological First aid

In 2009 the World Health Organization (WHO) recognised psychological first aid as valuable for reducing the physiological and psychological responses of people in severe distress provoked due to being exposed to trauma.

A guide developed by the Australian Red Cross and Australian Psychological Society (2013) defined psychological first aid as 'a humane, supportive and practical response to a person who has been exposed to serious stresses' and outlined its primary role as being to 'protect and promote the mental health and psychological wellbeing of survivors'.

Disaster recovery Psychologist Dr Rob Gordon (2004) suggests the following five elements for reducing arousal caused from exposure to a traumatic event:

1 Re-establishing a sense of physical safety;
2 Assisting survivors to reconnect with, or access information about, loved ones;
3 Helping survivors re-establish a sense of their needs;
4 Providing information and advice about reactions to help normalise their emotions; and
5 Providing information and advice about ways to promote recovery.

Helping a Client Manage Traumatic Stress

There are a number of strategies that can help a person resolve traumatic reactions.

- Recognise that you have been through a distressing or frightening experience and that you will have a reaction to it.
- Accept that you will not feel your normal self for a period of time, but that it will also eventually pass.
- Remind yourself daily that you are managing – try not to get angry or frustrated with yourself if you are not able to do things as well or efficiently as normal.
- Don't overuse alcohol or drugs to help you cope.
- Avoid making major decisions or big life changes until you feel better.

- Gradually confront what has happened – don't try to block it out.
- Don't bottle up your feelings – talk to someone who can support and understand you.
- Try to keep to your normal routine and stay busy.
- Don't go out of your way to avoid certain places or activities. Don't let the trauma confine your life, but take your time to get back to normal.
- When you feel exhausted, make sure you set aside time to rest.
- Make time for regular exercise – it helps cleanse your body and mind of tension.
- Help your family and friends to help you by telling them what you need, such as time out or someone to talk to.
- Relax – use relaxation techniques such as yoga, breathing or meditation, or do things you enjoy, such as listening to music or gardening.
- Express your feelings as they arise – talk to someone about your feelings or write them down.
- When the trauma brings up memories or feelings, try to confront them. Think about them, then put them aside. If it brings up other past memories, try to keep them separate from the current problem and deal with them separately.

(Better Health, 2022)

In Australia, there are various support services available to help people who have experienced trauma and trauma social workers will need to be aware of what support services are available in their area to resource and refer patients.

Post-traumatic Growth

As well as an awareness of the possible symptoms of acute traumatic stress, and an awareness of the psychosocial influences that can assist with recovery, working in the area of trauma requires an understanding of how the experience of traumatic injury and recovery can also have a positive influence on people. Calhoun and Tedeschi (2014) describe this as post-traumatic growth; they explain these changes in three general domains: 'changes in the perception of self, changes in the experience of relationships with others, and changes in one's general philosophy of life'. The human resilience they highlight is stated in first-person terms in this way: 'I am more vulnerable than I thought, but stronger than I ever imagined.'

Supporting Children Visiting the Intensive Care Unit

An easy oversight for hospital staff is to forget how daunting it can be for people visiting in the hospital environment; this is especially so when a family member or friend is seriously injured and placed in the intensive care unit (ICU). It can be even more challenging and emotional for children. Families are sometimes unsure or conflicted over whether children should be allowed to visit the ICU due to concern for the traumatic impact it may have on a child. The decision should be guided by the child's wishes along with the wishes of the family. Knutsson and Bergbom (2016) interviewed fourteen girls and fourteen boys around their experiences in ICU and stated:

> Children with a seriously ill/injured relative suffer. However, visiting seems to alleviate suffering. Visiting and being present as a part of the situation brought positive feelings of involvement and made it possible to show that they wanted to care for the

> relative. The sick relative was always on the child's mind and seeing and being with them in the intensive care unit resulted in relief and calmness, even if the relative's situation sometimes evoked feelings of despair and fear.

Trauma social workers can assist in this situation by supporting children and their family members during the visit. For example, the social worker can meet with the child prior to the visit to discuss how they are feeling, and can explain to the child the physical environment of ICU, and the purpose of the equipment attached to the patient. A doctor may also be happy to meet the child to explain the injuries. In the case of an unconscious patient, it may be valuable to advise the child that the patient's hand can be held, but the patient may not be able to respond. The child may like to take in a home-made card, or read to the patient from a favourite book. Ensure the child is aware that it's normal to be emotional, and if they feel distressed they can change their mind and leave at any time. Ensure they have a family member with them and support is available after the visit. Encourage them to talk about how they are feeling, and provide reassurance and normalise the emotions they may be experiencing.

Support to Individuals and Families Following a Suicide Attempt

A complex and sensitive issue requiring social work support is assistance for those affected by injury from self-harm or a suicide attempt. Patients can range from the very young to very old; the method of attempt can also vary, ranging from jumping from a height, hanging, knife injury, gun-shot wounds to transport-related accidents. The psychiatry team are referred to risk assess the patient's mental health and determine whether an inpatient psychiatric admission is required, or if community support is preferable to manage the person's mental health issues.

Alongside mental health issues, psychosocial issues can be a precipitating factor leading to self-injury. The role of the social worker can be to identify and provide support around any social issues that may be impacting. Studies have shown that younger people are more likely to self-harm (18–30 years), and that family problems and relationship issues are major precipitating factors (Ani et al., 2017; Devassy & Varghese, 2020). Precipitants can also differ across lifespans – such as middle-aged patients having fewer relationship issues, and younger patients having fewer financial and medical issues (Choo et al., 2018).

Close liaising with psychiatry and others involved from the multidisciplinary team is paramount in providing appropriate and effective support to the patient and their immediate social network. Due to the stigma of mental health and suicide it may be difficult for families to talk to others about the hospital admission. Families may have been concerned for the patient for a long time, they may have not known where to go for help; they may be feeling guilt that they were unable to prevent the suicide attempt. Sometimes the suicide can be completely unexpected and families struggle to find answers as to why this happened at all. Occasionally injuries are so severe the patient may have a permanent physical or cognitive impairment, or may even die as a result of their injuries.

On some occasions a child may have been a witness to the suicide attempt, and even gone to the person's aid. It is vital that children are provided with the help required to deal with this trauma. For school-aged children, ensure their school is aware so teachers and counsellors can support them. If required, a referral to a child mental health support service can be helpful in such situations. Families and friends may also seek advice on how to talk to the patient sensitively about the suicide attempt. Support and information on community resources are available on the internet that may be useful to the families.

End-of-Life/Bereavement Support

An emotionally sensitive time requiring social work support is assisting families through grief and loss and attending family meetings requiring end-of-life discussions. Medical staff may request a social worker's presence during this time to provide support, information and follow-up to families. In some circumstances these discussions may also involve conversations about organ donation. There are occasions when social workers are requested to be present and provide support to a patient when they are informed that someone has died or may die as a result of the same traumatic incident. In these situations it is important for medical staff to be aware and present during these discussions as the shock of the news may impact the patient medically. Providing information on grief and loss reactions and available supports is also valuable.

Providing Support after Injury as a Result of Family Violence

A hospital admission may be the first time a person has disclosed family violence; the hospital is therefore a critical area in providing sensitive and timely support to victims. A trauma patient may either have been admitted due to injury from a partner/family member, or during their admission it may come to light that domestic violence has been an ongoing issue and a risk issue for the person returning home. Family violence can be a very confronting and challenging intervention for social work; knowledge of the services available are necessary, as is training around supporting victims of family violence. Support may include assisting the person to find safe alternative housing, linking a patient with appropriate domestic violence services, liaising with police and providing a patient with legal advice and supportive counselling. Issues may also occur when a violent partner may attempt to visit the patient in hospital. Intervention should be guided by any legal orders and the patient's wishes, while at the same time giving consideration to their safety and vulnerability.

Child Protection

One of the more immediate responses required is to safeguard the welfare of a child or children if it comes to light they may be at risk of neglect or abuse. Issues regarding the safety and wellbeing of a child or children may be raised during any form of social work intervention, referrals may be made by medical staff, and occasionally from a child protection worker who may be aware of the hospital admission. Situations can arise where thoughtful balance is required between the need to report to child protection because child risk is suspected and protecting a person's privacy and their right for personal disclosures to be treated with confidentiality. The safety of the child is always paramount in such assessments and interventions. It is important to have a basic understanding of child protection legislation and mandatory reporting. When it is evident that a child is at risk, then child protection laws protect persons disclosing, and workplace policies provide guidance on how to respond in various situations.

Responding to Past Trauma

Trauma-informed practice is a framework that acknowledges the psychological impact of past adverse events. Having experienced past traumas can significantly impact upon a person during their hospital admission, awareness of this can enable the provision of appropriate support. Some patients may have psychological impacts from surviving physical and/or sexual abuse stemming as far back as childhood. Violently injured patients are disproportionately more likely to have a history of physical and psychological trauma (Fischer et al., 2019) and the immediate traumatic event and hospital admission may have a re-traumatising impact upon them.

Physical limitations caused by the recent injury, combined with the stress of being in the structured system of the hospital can be very challenging for some patients who in other situations would use strategies such as cigarettes, drugs and alcohol to cope with difficulties. When these are no longer accessible in the hospital environment the patient may find it very difficult to manage their frustration and emotions.

Fischer et al. (2019, p. 193) describe four pillars of trauma-informed care that they recommend in the delivery of care to patients with traumatic injuries:

- knowledge of the effect of trauma;
- recognition of the signs and symptoms of trauma;
- avoidance of re-traumatisation; and
- the development of appropriate policies and procedures.

A strength-based approach to explore past successful methods of coping can also be explored with the trauma patient.

Discharge Planning

Discharge planning is an integral part of working in trauma, and social workers alongside other allied health professionals such as physiotherapists and occupational therapists, play a key role in assisting patients with the transition from hospital to rehabilitation or home. Using the biopsychosocial model of health, social workers look at aspects of a patients' life to determine potential barriers and facilitators to discharge, such as the person's social supports, where they live, past experiences of trauma, and pre-existing or newly diagnosed mental health issues such as anxiety and depression.

Patients can leave hospital when they are medically safe, however they may not feel psychosocially ready. While most injured adults go on to experience a full recovery, a significant population develop psychiatric conditions such as PTSD and depression (Zatzick et al., 2011). An Australian study that followed up patients with significant trauma injuries for three years post hospital admission, found that just under half continued to experience anxiety/depression (Gabbe et al., 2017).

Social workers are instrumental in supporting the patients' wellbeing in hospital, and then linking the patient with the post-discharge supports necessary for patients with traumatic injuries to continue their psychological recovery.

Reflection: Bill's Story

Kathryn is an acute trauma social worker and was referred to see Bill who needed assistance with discharge planning. Bill was in his fifties and had been admitted to hospital after being violently assaulted by a resident in the boarding house where he lived. Kathryn was able to identify a potential barrier to discharge, when Bill told her he felt unsafe to return to the boarding house as he believed the person who had assaulted him still lived there; however, Bill had no other housing options.

Kathryn asked Bill if he had any past experiences with trauma. Bill replied that he had been sexually assaulted as a child and had grown up with a violent father. Both Bill's parents were now deceased, and he was no longer in touch with his siblings. Bill had married when younger and had two children, but he no longer had contact with his wife or children. Bill used drugs and alcohol daily, and acknowledged that this was to 'numb bad feelings'. He also talked of a longed-for future where he could afford to rent his own home and one day reconnect with his children who he had heard now had their own children.

Kathryn asked if he had any formal supports to help facilitate his return home. Bill replied that he had previously been assigned a housing officer, until he had been placed in the boarding house six months ago but had not heard from the officer since. Bill had previously tried counselling but had not found it terribly effective.

By liaising with police, Kathryn was able to establish that the person who had assaulted Bill was now remanded in custody and a protection order was in place preventing that resident returning to the boarding house, so Bill was safe to return there. With Bill's permission, Kathryn was able to contact his housing officer to explore longer term accommodation options. Kathryn also provided Bill with information on trauma and drug and alcohol support services given his history, and victims of crime services.

Reflection Questions

1 How much should Kathryn ask about Bill's childhood experiences?
2 What would be reasons for and against such exploration?
3 How would you integrate the practical aspects of discharge planning, with the psychological aspects of trauma counselling?

Other Single Session Supports

There are many reasons why the trauma social worker may be referred to. Assisting in practical issues can be a much-needed break from the emotionally intense support otherwise often required.

Legislation/Policy

It is recommended that social workers have a basic awareness and understanding of the following legislation areas specific to the state/country in which they are working, or know where to find the information when required (this list is not exhaustive):

- compensatory and legal entitlements;
- confidentiality/freedom of information;
- next of kin (specific laws vary between states);
- enduring power of attorney – a legal agreement that enables a person to appoint a trusted person or people to make financial and/or property decisions on their behalf;

- public health legislation;
- victims of crime;
- Mental Health Act;
- child protection;
- family violence.

Hospitals have policies and procedures as well as legal counsel that can be accessed when there is a need for advice on a complex situation.

Caring for Others

Occasionally a person's unplanned admission to a trauma ward leaves a person they care for at home, alone and vulnerable. Social workers can help by assessing how at risk the person home alone is, what support needs that person has, and exploring options for assisting such as other family/friends, or formal supports such as carer support services or residential respite. In the situation when the injured person is isolated and cares for a child or a young person with a disability, support from child protection may be required to find safe support until the patient is able to resume their carer role.

Media and Social Media

Some traumatic admissions can create interest in popular and social media, and journalists may attempt to speak with patients and families or friends for information and updates. Hospitals may have public affairs departments that families can be referred to; otherwise a social worker can provide some advice on how to manage such enquiries.

Communicating

Due to the sudden, unexpected nature of a trauma incident a patient may be admitted with no belonging, unidentified and no means of communicating with family and friends, social workers may be required to help identify and facilitate contact with next of kin and other relevant parties.

In the case of incidents with multiple casualties, including persons known to the patient, social workers may need to liaise with social work departments at other hospitals to establish communication and provide regular updates.

With the rise in the use of social media as a communication tool, social workers may be required to provide advice and support to patients and their significant others around safe use of social networking platforms to ensure accurate communication that is respectful of the patient's privacy.

Self-care

Working as a trauma social worker entails exposure to tragic circumstances, intense raw emotion, challenging behaviours, all while working in the highly bureaucratic, hierarchical, frequently changing structure of the hospital system. As Laurie Anne Pearlman, a clinical psychologist who has published and presented widely on psychological trauma, healing, and vicarious traumatisation, notes (Pearlman 2014):

> All of the trauma work that we do, hour after hour, day after day, week after week, contributes to inner changes in the self of the therapist. It's an inevitable part of the work … because we're entering into a very dark world, and if we're open emotionally, in the way we need to be to be effective helpers, we're going to be impacted.

It is important to understand the risk factors and the effects trauma social work can place on the social worker's mental health., and to regularly engage in activities that reduce stress, and seek support and to get help when impacted. Most health services will have employee support programmes, and social work departments provide regular supervision; in addition to the hospital, social workers can seek external supervision, psychology, and counselling.

Conclusion

Hospital-based trauma social work is intense and demanding, yet also very meaningful and rewarding in showing how connections and interventions can help people at points of crisis and distress. Whether it is responding to a physical injury or a mental health crisis, a suicide attempt, a death, domestic violence or homelessness, a social worker's day in this setting is unpredictable. It is important to remain focused on the work at hand, on the team and unit, on one's own self-care, and on the very real needs of the patients and families we serve.

Key Website Resources

Australian Red Cross (www.redcross.org.au/files/Psychological_First_Aid_An_Australian_Guide.pdf).

Better Health Channel: Trauma – Reaction and Recovery (www.betterhealth.vic.gov.au/health/conditionsandtreatments/trauma-reaction-and-recovery).

DSM V: http://dsm.psychiatryonline.org).

Victoria State Trauma System (www2.health.vic.gov.au/hospitals-and-health-services/patient-care/acute-care/state-trauma-system/major-trauma-classification).

References

AIHW. (2020). *National hospital morbidity database: findings based on unit record analysis.* Canberra: AIHW.

Ani, J. O., Ross, A. J. & Campbel, L. M. (2017). A review of patients presenting to accident and emergency department with deliberate self-harm, KwaZulu-Natal, South Africa. *African Journal of Primary Health Care and Family Medicine*, 9(1), 1–7.

Australian Red Cross and Australian Psychological Society. (2013). *Psychological first aid: an Australian guide to supporting people affected by disaster.* Australian Red Cross and Australian Psychological Society.

Better Health. (2022). Trauma – reaction and recovery. Retrieved from www.betterhealth.vic.gov.au/health/conditionsandtreatments/trauma-reaction-and-recovery.

Calhoun, L. G. & Tedeschi, R. G. (2014). *Handbook of posttraumatic growth: research and practice.* London: Routledge.

Choo C. C., Chew P. K. H. & Ho R. C. (2018). Suicide precipitants differ across the lifespan but are not significant in predicting medically severe attempts. *International Journal of Environmental Research and Public Health*, 15(4), 691. https://doi.org/10.3390/ijerph15040691.

Devassy, S. & Varghese, P. (2020). A cross-sectional study of the pattern of cases of deliberate self-harm in a tertiary care hospital. *Indian Journal of Forensic Medicine & Toxicology*, 14(3). doi:10.37506/ijfmt.v14i3.10333.

Fischer, K. R., Bakes, K. M., Corbin, T. J., Fein, J. A., Harris, E. J., James, T. L. & Melzer-Lange, M. D. (2019). Trauma-informed care for violently injured patients in the emergency department. *Annals of Emergency Medicine*, 73(2), 193–202.

Gabbe, B. J., Simpson, P. M., Cameron, P. A., Ponsford, J., Lyons, R. A., Collie, A., Fitzgerald, M., Judson, R., Teague, W. J., Braaf, S., Nunn, A., Ameratunga, S. & Harrison, J. E. (2017). Long-term health status and trajectories of seriously injured patients: A population-based longitudinal study. *PLOS Medicine*, 14, e1002322. doi:10.1371/journal.pmed.1002322.

Gordon, R. (2004). Community process and the recovery environment following emergency. *Environmental Health*, 4(1), 21–22.

Harris, D., Ellis, D. Y., Gorman, D., Foo, N. & Haustead, D. (2021). Impact of COVID-19 social restrictions on trauma presentations in South Australia. *Emergency medicine Australasia*, 33(1), 152–154.

Hoffman, G. R., Walton, G. M., Narelda, P., Qiu, M. M. & Alajami, A. (2020). COVID-19 Social distancing measures altered the epidemiology of facial injury: a UK–Australia comparative study. *The British Journal of Oral & Maxillofacial Surgery*, 59(4), 454–459.

Hopper, E.K., Bassuk, E.L. & Olivet, J. (2010). Shelter from the storm: trauma-informed care in homelessness services settings. *The Open Health Services and Policy Journal*, 3(2), 80–100.

Hugelius, K., Harada, N. & Marutani, M. (2021). Consequences of visiting restrictions during the COVID-19 pandemic: an integrative review. *International Journal of Nursing Studies*, 121, 104000.

Jacob, S., Mwagiru, D., Thakur, I., Moghadam, A., Oh, T. & Hsu, J. (2020). Impact of societal restrictions and lockdown on trauma admissions during the COVID-19 pandemic: a single-centre cross-sectional observational study. *ANZ Journal of Surgery*, 90(11), 2227–2231.

Kamine, T. H., Rembisz, A., Barron, R. J., Baldwin, C. & Kromer, M. (2020). Decrease in trauma admissions with COVID-19 pandemic. *Western Journal of Emergency Medicine*, 21(4), 819.

Knutsson, S. & Bergbom, I. (2016). Children's thoughts and feelings related to visiting critically ill relatives in an adult ICU: a qualitative study. *Intensive and Critical Care Nursing*, 32, 33–41.

Marques, R. R., Almeida, C. E., Coltro, P. S., Santos, L. A., Vecci, T. R. & Farina-Junior, J. A. (2021). Covid-19 pandemic has increased the incidence of self-inflicted burn injuries. *Burns*, 47 (8), 1931–1932.

McAlinden, F., McDermott, F. & Morris, J. (2013). Complex patients: social workers' perceptions of complexity in health and rehabilitation services. *Social Work in Health Care*, 52(10), 899–912.

McCann, I. L. & Pearlman, L. A. (1990). *Psychological trauma and the adult survivor: theory, therapy, and transformation.* New York: Brunner/Mazel.

Munshi, L., Evans, G. & Razak, F. (2021). The case for relaxing no-visitor policies in hospitals during the ongoing COVID-19 pandemic. *CMAJ*, 193(4), E135–E137.

Olding, J., Zisman, S., Olding, C. & Fan, K. (2021). Penetrating trauma during a global pandemic: changing patterns in interpersonal violence, self-harm and domestic violence in the Covid-19 outbreak. *The Surgeon*, 19(1), e9–e13.

Pearlman, L. A. (2014). *Vicarious traumatization.* Video file (approximately 86 minutes). San Francisco, CA: Kanopy Streaming.

Sayed, S., Iacoviello, B. M. & Charney, D. S. (2015). Risk factors for the development of psychopathology following trauma. *Current Psychiatry Reports*, 17(8), 1–7.

Silvera, G. A., Wolf, J. A., Stanowski, A. & Studer, Q. (2021). The influence of COVID-19 visitation restrictions on patient experience and safety outcomes: A critical role for subjective advocates. *Patient Experience Journal*, 8(1), 30–39.

Tedeschi, R. G. & Calhoun, L. G. (1995). *Trauma and transformation: growing in the aftermath of suffering.* Thousand Oaks, CA: Sage Publications.

Van Gelder, N., Peterman, A., Potts, A., O'Donnell, M., Thompson, K., Shah, N. & Oertelt-Prigione, S. (2020). COVID-19: Reducing the risk of infection might increase the risk of intimate partner violence. *EClinicalMedicine*, 21.

Veselsky, S. L., Poirier, M. V., Tracy, B. M., Castater, C. A., Mehta, C., Minihan, A. K., Williams, K. N., Gelbard, R. B., Faloye, A. O. & Smith, R. N. (2021). Mechanisms of self-inflicted injuries at an urban city hospital. *The American Surgeon*, 88(7), 1669–1674.

Waseem, S., Nayar, S. K., Hull, P., Carrothers, A., Rawal, J., Chou, D. & Khanduja, V. (2021). The global burden of trauma during the COVID-19 pandemic: a scoping review. *Journal of Clinical Orthopaedics and Trauma*, 12(1), 200–207.

Zatzick, D., Rivara, F., Jurkovich, G., Russo, J., Trusz, S. G., Wang, J. & Petrie, M. (2011). Enhancing the population impact of collaborative care interventions: mixed method development and implementation of stepped care targeting posttraumatic stress disorder and related comorbidities after acute trauma. *General Hospital Psychiatry*, 3(2), 123–134.

6 Mental Health Social Work

Recovery-Oriented Practice Engagement and Collaboration

Jacinta Chavulak, Kate Day and Melissa Petrakis

Introduction

Social workers play a key role in supporting people who experience mental health issues, regardless of the service they work in. It is useful for all social workers to be aware of best practice working with people who experience mental health issues, in order to support mental wellness. Most recent Australian statistics indicate that 1 in 5 people (20%, or 4.8 million) reported a mental and/or behaviour condition in the previous 12 months (Australian Institute of Health and Wellbeing 2020). This chapter explores theory underpinning practice by providing an overview of frameworks for practice and explores mental health legislation in Australia and internationally. It also provides an overview of how to assess and intervene when working with people with mental health issues. It provides an overview of diagnoses experienced by people, exploring both low and high prevalence disorders. Throughout the chapter there are examples provided of models commonly used within the mental health field. Across all of these domains we will endeavour to highlight some of the ethical issues that arise in mental health social work. Raising these ethical issues will encourage you to consider critical approaches to social work and their application. All authors have worked in mental health direct practice which informs this chapter.

Frameworks for Practice

Three key models for working in mental health are *early intervention, recovery-orientated practice* and *strengths-based approach*, as well as legislation in which social work interventions are bound by, are explored below.

Early Intervention

In the early 1990s early intervention in psychosis started to emerge as a model for best practice (Falloon 1992). Since this time early intervention has become well-established approach, which is funded and included in the mainstream mental health system (Killackey & Yung 2007).

Advocates for early intervention contend that this approach improves the prognosis for people who are diagnosed with a psychotic disorder (McGorry 2005). There is a strong argument contending that reducing the duration of untreated psychosis improves the prognosis for people early in the course of a psychotic illness (Killackey & Yung 2007).

Key principles for early intervention:

DOI: 10.4324/9781003330745-8

- Early intervention can delay the onset of psychosis and improve the prognosis for those who have experienced psychosis.
- Ease of access to services is paramount.
- A biopsychosocial approach should be employed.
- The stage of illness is important and must be considered when providing treatment.
- Services should be inclusive of family members or significant others.

(Early Psychosis Guidelines Writing Group 2010)

Recovery Orientated Practice

'Recovery' has been described as 'a consistent unifying principle in contemporary mental health policies and services' (Bland et al. 2009, p. 43). This principal gained traction in the 1990's after the creation of a community based service system to replace psychiatric institutions had proved extremely difficult: it became clear that a fundamental paradigm shift was required to meet the needs of people with mental ill health in a community setting (Anthony 1993). Recovery upholds the belief that people with a mental illness can have meaningful and productive lives, regardless of whether full symptom remission is achieved. In this paradigm, personal experience is greatly valued and self-determination is integral. The recovery movement has been led by service users of mental health services who are demanding to occupy space within the system where they can contribute to decision-making processes and ensure that their rights are upheld.

A systematic review published in the *British Journal of Psychiatry* provides an excellent explanation of recovery (Leamy et al. 2011). This review examines published descriptions and models of recovery with the aim of drawing together commonalities. The review situates recovery-based practice at the core of mental health service provision as an empirically supported approach that needs to be genuinely pursued by clinicians and supported by service providers. Further, the review provides some conceptual clarity around recovery, including the identification of five common recovery processes, making up the acronym CHIME:

- Connectedness;
- Hope and optimism about the future;
- Identity;
- Meaning in life; and
- Empowerment.

In Australia the Framework for Recovery Oriented Practice has been created as part of The National Mental Health Strategy (Mental Health Drug and Alcohol Principal Committee 2013). This framework provides some guidance to practitioners and services around how best to provide recovery-based interventions. Five domains that provide the foundation for service provision are identified. They are:

- Promoting a culture and language of hope and optimism.
- Person first and holistic.
- Supporting personal recovery.
- Organisational commitment and workforce development
- Action on social inclusion and the social determinants of health, mental health and wellbeing.

Strengths-Based Approach

The strengths model has developed alongside the recovery movement and provides one formula for recovery-orientated practice (Petrakis et al. 2014). The model is outlined in Rapp and Gosha's *The Strengths Model* (2011). Like recovery, this model demands that mental illness is viewed through a different lens. It assertively provides an alternative to the medical model for understanding and treating mental illness: the focus on strengths challenges the conventional focus on deficits and pathologies. The model describes the social, occupational, recreational and relationship pursuits of individuals as the 'personal medicine' that contributes to recovery and creates meaning in people's lives (Rapp & Goscha 2011 p. 19). The model explicitly states that recovery does not mean an absence of symptoms and is openly critical of the incumbent system of care that has typically pursued this end. Clinicians are asked to find 'hope inducing practices' and work alongside service users to combat 'spirit-crushing' circumstances within society, such as poverty and stigma, or practices within the system of care (Rapp & Goscha 2011). A recent review examining a modest number of studies on strengths based mental health interventions concluded that this approach has a growing evidence base. Outcomes suggested to be associated with the use of this model included reduced hospitalisation rates and improved occupational and relationship outcomes (Tse et al. 2016).

The strengths model has been operationalised to varying degrees and employed by a number of mental health service providers across Australia. The model fits well with early intervention's focus on reducing the impact of developing a psychotic illness on the developmental trajectory of people who develop a psychotic illness and promoting social recovery.

Involuntary Treatment and a Rights-Based Approach

Like many areas of social work practice, mental health practice is closely tied to a legislative framework. Contemporary mental health legislation has the difficult role of defining the circumstances and boundaries of involuntary treatment while at the same time protecting the human rights, self-determination and dignity of mental health service users. Mental health clinicians are often involved in placing people under involuntary treatment, and work with people who are currently under involuntary treatment. This places social workers in an ethical mine field where our social work values of promoting autonomy and self-determination are challenged by the need to ensure safety by enacting involuntary treatment. Some Social Workers reject the notion that Social Workers should be engaging in enacting involuntary treatment orders and it is not aligned with Social Work values (Maylea, 2017). For this reason it is crucially important that our practice is informed by human rights principles. In 2006, 164 countries were signatories for The Convention on the Rights of Persons with Disabilities (CRPD), which outlines fundamental human rights for those with a disability, which also includes those with a mental illness (United Nations 2006). It promotes principles of dignity, respect and equality, and signatories have committed to ensuring the freedom from torture or degrading treatment. This document is integral to consider when reflecting on the use of involuntary treatment for people with mental illness.

In Australia (a signatory of the CRPD), National Mental Health Policy (Department of Health 2008) guides best practice in this field, which is currently under review (with a proposed 2021–2022 roadmap currently in action at time of publication). Recovery-orientated practice is embedded in this document, with a key directive for early intervention and autonomy within treatment options. These are key principles, however can become difficult to enact under current systems of involuntary treatment.

There have been efforts throughout Australia and internationally to move away from outdated, restrictive and paternalistic models and create a framework that is more aligned with recovery-orientated approaches. For example, there is currently a review of the Mental Health Act Victoria (2014). This philosophical shift include promotion of individual's rights and autonomy and the need for treatment to be in the least restrictive environment among its core principles. There have been changes to the procedure around providing involuntary treatment and these changes generally represent a shift towards greater autonomy for service users.

Involuntary treatment is enacted if a person is believed to have a mental illness that requires immediate treatment to prevent them from serious deterioration of their physical or mental health or serious harm to the person or to another person. In these circumstances a legal order can be put in place requiring them to have compulsory treatment (Health Victoria 2014). Depending on the location, the specific terms of this changes, treatment usually involves medication and potentially involuntary admission to a psychiatric hospital. While in hospital, a patient might also experience restrictive interventions (medical, mechanical and/or physical restraint, as well as periods of seclusion). Efforts are being made to reduce restrictive interventions, however these are still widely practised across Australia and internationally (Chavulak & Petrakis 2017).

Reflection

The different frameworks for practice that we draw from in this area can be seen as presenting us with a number of competing demands. For example, early psychosis guidelines require us to carefully assess the positive symptoms of psychosis to guide treatment, whereas the strengths model asks us to move away from a pathologising focus on symptomology. Similarly, and perhaps more starkly, the recovery movement promotes people within the mental health system having a greater degree of self-determination while the Mental Health Act provides clinicians with the power treat service users involuntarily in certain circumstances.

Reflection Questions

1. What are some strategies that you could use to reconcile the ideological and practical differences between these practice frameworks?
2. What can you as a social work practitioner do in a clinical mental health setting to redress the power imbalance that unavoidable under legislation giving clinicians the power to treat people involuntarily? How might you use the other frameworks outlined above in doing so?

Diagnoses and Symptoms

Social workers are required to have an understanding of the types of mental health diagnoses that are utilised to inform treatment plans. Whether social workers are working directly in mental health services, or working in different service sectors, it is useful to understand what cluster of symptoms form specific diagnoses. While every person is unique, and their illnesses may present differently, it's useful to have an understanding of how mental health issues may affect their presentation, and how one might be best supported.

Diagnoses are a key tool of the medical model which social workers will need to work within in some contexts (for example, if you work in a clinical mental health team as outlined in the following chapter). A diagnosis does not provide a full picture of what an individual experiences, a diagnosis is a labelling tool to inform treatment. Each individual will experience a diagnosis differently, and it is important to explore how people you will work with understand their own diagnosis and what it means to them.

The Diagnostic and Statistical Manual of Mental Disorders (DSM-5) is the handbook utilised in Australia (and internationally) to categorise types of mental health issues people experience. A mental disorder is defined by the DSM-5 as 'a syndrome characterized by clinically significant disturbance in an individual's cognition or behaviour that reflects a dysfunction in the psychological, biological, or developments processes underlying mental functioning' (American Psychiatric Association 2013, p. 20). This definition highlights the importance of a biopsychosocial assessment within the medical model, demonstrating social work's key role within the mental health system. A useful text to further your understanding of working within this field is *Social Work Practice in Mental Health: An Introduction* (Bland et al. 2009). More common disorders (high prevalence disorders) include anxiety and depressive disorders. Less common disorders (low prevalence disorders) include disorders involving psychosis such as schizophrenia and bipolar affective disorder. Personality disorders affect a person's behaviour not fitting with cultural norms will also be explored. This section is a brief overview only and you are encouraged to read more widely to further to knowledge to support you in the field.

High-Prevalence Mental Health Disorders

Everyone will experience feelings of anxiety or sadness across their lifetime, however in order for someone to meet the criteria for a diagnosis for a mental health disorder, a more enduring and severe experience occurs, and these have a significant impact on their ability to participate in life.

Depression

Depressive disorders involve a pervasive low mood (e.g. sad, irritable, flat) with impaired cognitive functioning (e.g. foggy thoughts, impaired memory, difficulty making decisions) and activities of daily living (e.g. being able to wash, eat, dress, leave the house, go to work/study).

Anxiety

Anxiety disorders are a group of disorders which include a feelings of fear, intrusive thoughts, difficulty with cognition, and physical disturbances such as nausea, sweating and panic attacks. Generalised anxiety disorder, panic disorder and phobias are all types of anxiety disorders.

Depending on the severity of the disorder, medication may be needed. However activities such as exercise, a good diet, a good routine, social connection and meaningful activity is often utilised to help treat these disorders.

Low-Prevalence Mental Health Disorders

This chapter focuses more on working with people who have experienced an episode of psychosis, so further detail will be provided in order to inform practice.

Psychosis

Psychosis is a group of symptoms, if one or more of these symptoms are experienced over a period of time, a person may be diagnosed with a psychotic illness explored below.

Five key features of psychotic disorders are explored below as per DSM-5:

1. Delusions – a non-reality based strong belief not fitting with cultural norms. Examples include believing the government is listening or watching or that the person experiencing the delusion is a God-like figure.
2. Hallucinations – a perceptual disturbance: seeing, feeling, smelling, tasting or hearing something without the correlating stimuli. Examples are hearing voices (most common) or feeling sensations on the body without being touched.
3. Disorganised thinking – referred to as thought disorder, where the form of the thoughts are mixed up. Examples are: switching from one topic or word without association, nonsensical speech.
4. Behavioural problems – abnormal motor behaviour. Examples include the body becoming motionless and becoming verbally non-responsive.
5. Negative symptoms – loss of normal brain function, similar to a depressive state. Examples include a sense of emotional numbness and unable to enjoy usual activities.

Schizophrenia

Schizophrenia is a psychotic disorder, where two of the five symptoms outlined previously are experienced for a significant amount of time for a period of four weeks, coupled with a marked decline in functioning for the past six months. These symptoms are not rapidly fluctuating (or a delirium might be considered) or dependent on stressful circumstances (or a personality disorder might be considered). There are related psychotic disorders which may be diagnosed (such as schizoaffective disorder, which has a mood component).

Bipolar Disorder

Bipolar affective disorder (BPAD) is a mood disorder, one with quite severe shifts in mood which often results in experiencing psychosis. The mood shifts are extreme in nature, from depressive episodes (characterised by low mood, lack of motivation, changes in appetite and sleep, limited enjoyment in daily life) to manic episodes (elevated mood, delusions of grandeur, increase in risk taking behaviours, excessive and compulsive high stimulus activities such as spending, gambling, sexual activities). There are different types of BPAD, with varying degrees of mood and manic episodes. A key feature of this disorder is that the episodes last a period of time (e.g. the changes are not over hours or days, but rather weeks and months).

Treatment for high prevalence disorders includes medication, therapy, connection to meaningful activities and support through stressful life circumstances (such as ensuring appropriate housing).

Personality Disorders

Personality disorders are a pattern of internal experiences which severely affect behaviour, often whereby internal distress is externalised. Personality disorders are a cluster of disorders outlined in the DSM-5, and are grouped into three sections: where the person's personality is odd, intensely emotional or anxious. A common personality disorder is borderline personality disorder, which involves a fluctuating sense of self, difficulty regulating emotions, marked impulsivity, often engaging in self injurious behaviours and difficulty in interpersonal relationships. Someone with a diagnosis of a personality disorder may experience a psychotic episode, however it is not a key component in the diagnosis. Often these episodes are related to significant trauma which has been linked to the development of personality disorders (Perry & Lee 2020). There is significant stigma associated with personality disorders; many believe the terms (and often treatments) are not appropriate for those who have experienced significant trauma and have petitioned for them to be revised (Van der Kolk 2015). Treatment for personality disorders varies, and medication may be required to manage symptoms of acute distress in early phases of recovery, however structured and tailored therapy with access to crisis containment is currently recommended.

All mental disorders can improve over time, and utilising a recovery-orientated approach, social workers can support recovery journeys by ensuring that the person is involved in decisions about their treatment, that support is tailored to the needs of the individual and that an individual's strength are recognised and genuinely utilised throughout the process. It is important to recognise the episodic nature of mental health issues, and that times of being unwell can be reduced, managed and improved over time. Recovery does not mean living without symptoms, but living a meaningful life.

Reflection

Clinical mental health is traditionally a field dominated by the medical model. However, overtime more voices are being included in the discourse of mental health. Social work is one area that is contributing to this greater diversity and social work interventions in mental health are certainly common. However, the medical approach to research and evidence continues to be dominant. Social work approaches to research may be more flexible and inclusive.

Reflection Questions

1 Can you identify some parallels between approaches to practice and approaches to research?
2 How could viewing these issues through a social work lens and value to the current state of research in Mental health?
3 What is the nature of evidence required for a practice to be considered as 'evidence-based'?
4 Are there different types of evidence that might be helpful in this field and how could they contribute to our knowledge base and the field?

Assessment and Interventions

Clinical mental health services traditionally work within the structure of a medical hierarchy and social workers can at times find this challenging. The focus can be on mitigating risk and alleviating symptoms with the use of anti-psychotic medications while addressing the more intangible social situation of service users can take second place. While it is important that mental health social workers develop an understanding of the medical approach to managing mental health, our developing understanding of recovery suggests that while remission of symptoms is desirable the process of social and functional recovery is just as important (Early Psychosis Guidelines Writing Group 2010; Leamy et al. 2011). Before undertaking an assessment it is important, if possible, to gather any collateral information that may be relevant. This could include discharge summaries from previous services, or contact with the parents of a young person.

Biopsychosocial Assessment Approach

Assessments should take a biopsychosocial approach (Bland et al. 2009; AASW 2014). This is especially important in early intervention because all of the different spheres provide important context that inform the direction that treatment should take. Assessments should include a discussion of family and medical history, occupational functioning, social situation including housing, relationships and supports, and psychological functioning, for example coping strategies. These assessments should also include an exploration of the person's strengths and attributes and avoid a narrow focus on psychopathology.

Mental State Examination

Mental state examination (MSE) is an assessment of signs and symptoms of a mental disorder. This includes making observations about the person's appearance, speech, mood and behaviour, an assessment of their thinking in terms of content and cohesiveness, an account of any evidence or reports of distorted perceptions such as auditory hallucinations and the person's cognitive functioning. An MSE should also note the person's own understanding of their situation and their ability to make sound judgements. An MSE should be a part of an initial assessment but also undertaken regularly.

Risk

Risk assessment is an important part of both initial assessment and ongoing assessment. However, assessing risk should not dominate the assessment. Areas of risk that need to be considered include: risk of suicidality, risk to others, risk of vulnerability, risk to physical health, risk of deterioration in mental health and risk to reputation. Some of these risks may be immediate and would require action, perhaps under the Mental Health Act, whereas other risks may be longer term and require ongoing conversations with the person. A risk assessment should also include details about any protective factors that may mitigate risk, for example strong family support.

Interventions and Ongoing Treatment

Based on your initial assessment and in collaboration with the person you will need to identify the type of interventions that might be useful in each situation. The most important factor in making these decisions is the stage of illness of the person. A person who is in crisis, with ongoing positive psychotic symptoms and currently in an inpatient unit, will have very different needs from someone living in the community, going to work or school and trying to manage their own medication.

Psychoeducation: Making Sense of the Experience

Social workers support people to make sense of the experience that they have had. It involves providing a safe space in which to reflect on their experience, providing information about psychosis in small portions when this relevant to the person and coming to an explanation of what has happened that is acceptable to the person.

There are some useful tools that can be used to provide information to people and their families. These particular tools will have some relevance to most people.

The 'stress vulnerability' model is based on the premise that every person is vulnerable to psychosis given a particular set of circumstances (Zubin & Spring 1977). This model outlines a number of factors that can contribute to a person becoming psychotic, the combination of factors that lead to a person becoming psychotic are unique to each individual (Figure 6.1). This model supports the idea that it is the interaction between a person's genetic make-up and their environment that contributes to mental ill health.

The 'phases of recovery' model, developed by Orygen Youth Health (Yung & McGorry 1996), provides people with some idea of how their recovery may progress. The model shows that before becoming unwell most people will have a prodromal period; during this period people may experience low-grade psychotic symptoms and functional decline (Figure 6.2). Some people will then go on to become acutely unwell, after which there will be an early recovery stage during which people usually improve quite rapidly.

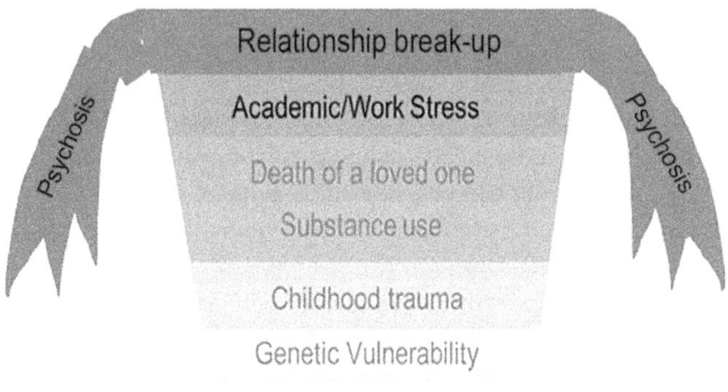

Figure 6.1 The stress vulnerability model

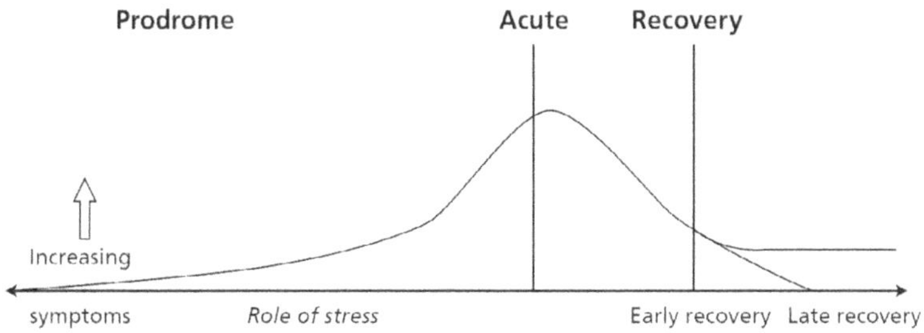

Figure 6.2 Phases of recovery model

The final stage described by this model is the late recovery stage. This stage may last for many months, which is usually longer than people expect, during this time people may continue to be at a lower level of functioning, lack motivation and become depressed all of which can be extremely frustrating. It is helpful for clinicians to discuss this with people, normalise the experience of having a protracted recovery stage and foster hope that recovery will continue.

Relapse Prevention

After someone has had a psychotic experience the likelihood that they will go on to have a relapse at some stage is quite high. Given this it is important to engage in planning around relapse prevention. This should be framed in a hopeful way rather than pessimistic way and couched in a broader conversation about recovery. For example, we can give people the message that recovery is expected, that it means different things for different people, and that planning for how best to manage relapse may help to avoid it altogether or significantly reduce its impact if it does occur.

Relapse prevention work can follow on very well from supporting people to make sense of their experience. An in-depth exploration of the symptoms that people experienced when becoming unwell provides the basis for good relapse prevention planning (Birchwood et al. 2000). Having these conversations with people while they are well creates a strong foundation for the work that we do with people when they become unwell. Creating written plans with people is a key part of this process and these documents provide a tangible agreement to refer back to.

Medication

When starting in the field of mental health most social workers will identify learning about psychotropic medications as one of their greatest challenges. However, it is important that we develop a basic knowledge of relevant medication to inform our practice and assist us to support the people that we work with.

There are three main types of medication that we will come across. These are anti-psychotic medications, mood stabilisers and anti-depressants. The relationship that people have with these medications is extremely complex. There are all sorts of reasons that people may not take their medication as prescribed and giving people the opportunity to have transparent discussions about this is an important part of our role. These conversations are often integral to other interventions, such as relapse prevention. Most medications have side effects, which can have severe impacts on someone's quality of life. It is important to ensure that someone is on the lowest possible therapeutic dose of medication to reduce this risk. It is also useful to explore alternative medications if side effects are experienced. We can further support people with this part of their treatment by maintaining the principles of shared decision making (Simmons et al. 2012).

Metabolic Monitoring

Many medications, antipsychotics in particular, can cause people who take them to develop side effects such as significant weight gain, problems with metabolising sugars and hypotension; a combination of these symptoms is referred to as metabolic syndrome. Weight, waist circumference, blood pressure and blood tests are reviewed regularly. This is especially important when they start on a new medication. As mental health social workers are often people's primary contact at the mental health service and we have an ongoing relationship with them, it is important that we, along with other clinicians, take responsibility for monitoring people's physical health and supporting them to address their health needs. It is important to consider other risks associated with this intervention and be sensitive, for example, those who experience eating disorders may find this extremely distressing. As usual, involving people in their own care is integral to a therapeutic intervention.

Reflection: Sam's Story

You are working in a youth drop-in centre and you notice one of the regular young people who access the service is acting differently. Sam is a 21-year-old woman who has had a trauma history and experiences homelessness. She is usually bright, reactive, engaged in activities and friendly. Today she is appearing agitated and has had an argument with another service user. She is refusing food as they believe it is poisoned. She is not known to be a substance user, however you notice her pupils are dilated and she appears on edge and fidgety. Her clothes are torn and dirty, however she usually prides herself on her presentation and fashion is an important part of her self-expression. She does not have a history of psychosis or a diagnosed mental illness, however has reported previously feelings of sadness and worry which have been linked to stressors in her life.

Key Practice Questions

1. Conduct a mental state examination – what are some indicators that the young person may be experiencing mental health issues? What questions would you ask to obtain more information?
2. Conduct a risk assessment – what are the key risk factors that need to be mitigated?
3. What steps could you take to mitigate the risks outlined above?
4. What are some referrals that may be useful for ongoing support?

Conclusion

This chapter has provided an overview of working with people with mental health issues. This importance of intervening early has been outlined, the role that social workers play, and the importance of this role, has been discussed. Many of the interventions and practices described here will be relevant to social work in mental health more broadly, however, social workers must always be conscious when working in mental health that the way we practice will form an important part of their understanding of and feelings towards the service system, as well as supporting them in their own, unique recovery.

Key Website Resources

International Early Psychosis Association (IEPA) (https://iepa.org.au). IEPA is an international network for those involved in the study and treatment of the early phases of mental health disorders and includes resources for service users and families.

Early Psychosis Prevention and Intervention Centre (EPPIC) (http://oyh.org.au). Centre for research and innovation in early psychosis. The organisation provides accessible information about early psychosis that is relevant to practitioners, young people and their family members and friends.

Early Intervention in Psychiatry (journal) (http://onlinelibrary.wiley.com/journal/10.1111/(ISSN)1751-7893). The official journal of the IEPA Early Intervention in Mental Health Inc.

Understanding psychosis – for health professionals (http://headspace.org.au/health-professionals/understanding-psychosis-for-health-professionals). Headspace in Australia has provided easily accessible information for professionals who work with young people, and anyone else who is looking for details of existing research in youth mental health.

References

American Psychiatric Association. (2013) *Diagnostic and Statistical Manual of Mental Disorders* (5th ed.). Washington, DC: American Psychiatric Association.

Anthony, W. (1993) Recovery from mental illness: the guiding vision of the mental health service system in the 1990s. *Psychosocial Rehabilitation Journal* 16(4): 11–23.

Australian Association of Social Workers. (2014) *Practice Standards for Mental Health Social Workers 2014*. Canberra: Australian Association of Social Workers.

Australian Institute of Health and Wellbeing. (2020) Report on mental health. Retrieved from www.aihw.gov.au/reports/australias-health/mental-health.

Birchwood, M., E. Spencer & D. McGovern (2000) Schizophrenia: early warning signs. *Advances in Psychiatric Treatment* 6: 33–101.

Bland, R., N. Renouf & A. Tullgren (2009) *Social Work Practice in Mental Health: An Introduction*. Crows Nest, NSW: Allen & Unwin.

Chavulak, J. & M. Petrakis. (2017) Who experiences seclusion? An examination of demographics and duration in a public acute inpatient mental health service. *Social Work in Health Care* 56(6): 524–540.

Department of Health. (2008) National mental health policy. Retrieved from www.health.gov.au/resources/publications/national-mental-health-policy-2008.

Department of Health. (2010) National standards for mental health services. Retrieved from www.health.gov.au/sites/default/files/documents/2021/04/national-standards-for-mental-health-services-2010-and-implementation-guidelines-national-standards-for-mental-health-services-2010.pdf.

Department of Health & Human Services. (2013) Framework for reducing restrictive interventions. Retrieved from www2.health.vic.gov.au/mental-health/practice-and-service-quality/safety/reducing-restrictive-interventions/framework-for-reducing-restrictive-interventions.

Early Psychosis Guidelines Writing Group. (2010) *Australian Clinical Guidelines for Early Psychosis*. Melbourne: Orygen Youth Health.

Falloon, I. R. H. (1992) Early intervention for first episodes of schizophrenia: a preliminary exploration. *Psychiatry* 55: 4–15.

Health Victoria. (2014) Mental Health Act 2014 handbook. Retrieved from www2.health.vic.gov.au/mental-health/practice-and-service-quality/mental-health-act-2014-handbook.

Killackey, E. & A. Yung. (2007) Effectiveness of early intervention in psychosis. *Current Opinion Psychiatry* 20: 121–125.

Leamy, M., V. Bird, C. Le Boutillier, J. Williams & M. Slade. (2011) Conceptual framework for personal recovery in mental health: systematic review and narrative synthesis. *British Journal of Psychiatry* 199: 445–452.

Maylea, C. H. (2017) A rejection of involuntary treatment in mental health social work. *Ethics and Social Welfare* 11(4): 336–352.

McGorry, P. (2005) Early intervention in psychotic disorders: beyond debate to solving problems. *British Journal of Psychiatry* 187: 108–110.

Mental Health Drug and Alcohol Principal Committee. (2013) *A National Framework for Recovery-Oriented Mental Health Services: Guide for Practitioners and Providers*. Canberra: Department of Health and Aging.

Perry, C. & R. Lee (2020) Childhood trauma and personality disorder. In G. Spalletta *et al.* (eds), *Childhood Trauma in Mental Disorders*. Cham: Springer.

Petrakis, M., H. Bloom & J. Oxley. (2014) Family perceptions of benefits and barriers to first episode psychosis carer group participation. *Social Work in Mental Health* 12(2): 99–116.

Rapp, C. A. & R. J. Goscha. (2011) *The Strengths Model: A Recovery Oriented Approach to Mental Health Services*. New York: Oxford University Press.

Simmons, M., S. Rice, S. Hetrick, A. Bailey & A. Parker. (2012) *Shared Decision Making (SDM) for Mental Health: What is the Evidence?*O. Y. H. R. Centre.

Tse, S., E. W. S. Tsoi, B. Hamilton, M. O'Hagan, G. Shepherd, M. Slade, R. Whitley & M. Petrakis. (2016) Use of strength-based interventions for people with serious mental illness: a critical review. *International Journal of Social Psychiatry* 62(3): 281–291.

United Nations. (2006) *The Convention on the Rights of Persons with Disabilities*. New York: United Nations.

Van der Kolk, B. A. (2015) *The Body Keeps the Score: Brain, Mind, and Body in the Healing of Trauma*. New York: Penguin Books.

Yung, A. & P. McGorry. (1996) The prodromal phase of first-episode psychosis: past and current conceptualizations. *Schizophrenia Bulletin* 22(2): 353–370.

Zubin, J. & B. Spring (1977) Vulnerability: a new view of schizophrenia. *Journal of Abnormal Psychology* 86(2): 103–126.

7 Social Work Advanced Practice Skills in Mental Health

Carmel Alakus, Jacinta Chavulak and Melissa Petrakis

Introduction

This chapter aims to develop advanced skills required of social workers employed in the mental health field. It provides an historical context for practice and outlines how changes to mental health services impact service delivery. It describes some current mental health service systems both in Australia and Internationally. The social work role in mental health is thoroughly explored, detailing specific tasks performed. For social work students considering a future in clinical mental health, strategies for surviving and thriving are discussed in the context of enhancing social work practice more broadly.

Historical Reflection: Clinical Mental Health Services since Deinstitutionalisation

Since the late 1950s there has been an international shift regarding the way mental health services have been delivered (Shen & Snowden, 2014). Both the World Health Organization (WHO) and United Nations (UN) have supported a shift to deinstitutionalisation and have policies exploring the same. Deinstitutionalisation can be defined as 'a policy that mandates a shift in practice of caring for individuals with mental illness from institutional environments to the community' (Shen & Snowden, 2014, p. 1). This process has varied internationally, with some countries still working through this process today. Since closing larger psychiatric hospitals, acute psychiatric in-patient care is mostly now provided by local hospitals, with community based mental health teams and, in some cases, dedicated mental health accommodation is provided by government and non-government organisations. The enormous advantages of deinstitutionalisation meant that people can receive a service in their locality and that psychiatric services can be more in touch and responsive to their communities. They tend to be seen as more humane and responding to people's individual needs and are more cost effective (Shen & Snowden, 2014).

A non-systematic trend towards deinstitutionalisation occurred from the 1950s assisted by clinical optimism, availability of employment and changing social attitudes (Rosen, 2006). During the 1970–1980s some community health teams were put in place throughout the developed world, but they typically focused idealistically on primary prevention, and typically were generic rather than specialist in nature.

Deinstitutionalisation is also referred to as *integration* in the First National Mental Health Plan (1993–1998). It came about in Victoria in Australia, where the authors are based, in the 1990s (Human Services Victoria Mental Health Branch, 1994). Area Mental Health Services

DOI: 10.4324/9781003330745-9

were developed which included the introduction of Crisis Assessment and Treatment Teams (CATT), case management teams called Continuing Care Teams (CCT) and specialised mid-term accommodation with clinical support called Continuing Care Units (CCUs).

Although there have been many positive gains from de-institutionalisation, including tailored care and overall commitment to service user rights, there has been criticism. Housing services, nationally, many of which employ social workers, tell another side to the story. When the larger psychiatric hospitals or 'asylums' were closed, so did the option for mid-long term psychiatric admissions. Some service users reported mixed responses to this (Leggatt & Jeffs, 2020). There simply was not enough housing stock to meet the special needs of people diagnosed with serious mental illness, resulting in many being placed in transitional housing, rooming houses or accommodation that did not sufficiently meet their needs. Families and carers were expected to assume a greater responsibility of care. All of this led to a lower quality of life and poor long-term outcomes for some (Papakotsias & Zimmerman, 2012).

Practice Implications: Current Mental Health Practice

Services vary depending on where social workers practice. This section explores different types of services mental health social workers are employed in and what role they play. Of note, the unequal distribution of resources across the planet impacts service delivery, and services from low or middle resourced countries tend to continue to have a hospital-based focus. However there has been global improvement over the last decade (Saxena et al, 2019). Efforts have been made by international bodies to create more accessible community based mental health services, however this continues to be impacted by economic, historical and cultural contexts (Shen & Snowden, 2014; Saxena et al., 2019). There has been a global push towards a human rights-based approach to mental health care, which aligns with social work values (Austin, 2017; Australian Association of Social Workers, 2010). The following is a general overview of types of mental health services, written by experienced clinicians located in Victoria, Australia.

Clinical Mental Health Services

In-patient Admissions

In-patient admissions often involve shorter stays with a focus on providing support during an acute mental health episode, with follow-up treatment occurring in the community. During an in-patient episode, social workers on psychiatric wards assist patients by ensuring they have economic support (this may involve making application for income support or welfare payments) and somewhere to live on discharge (this may involve linking them to a housing services). The social worker is routinely involved in formulating treatment plans (this may involve joining in clinical discussion meetings with nursing and medical staff including their treating psychiatrist.) Finally, the social worker assists with any other psycho-social issues for which service users may need additional support.

Crisis Support

There is an acknowledgement that mental health issues are episodic in nature and may not require long term clinical support. For episodes of acute mental distress, community-based crisis teams can respond to provide swift support. This may involve providing medical reviews by a psychiatrist, monitoring risk and mental state, and linking people to longer term supports if needed. This type of care could be viewed as a 'hospital in the home' arrangement. Social Workers are often employed alongside other mental health clinicians and provide insight and reflection within a traditionally medical model intervention. Social workers are integral in developing treatment plans, in developing formulations and guiding interventions which best support people in a time of crisis.

Community-Based Support

This is often referred to as 'case management' and involves allocating a mental health clinician to an individual (and their families) to support them living with a severe and persistent mental illness. Support is provided mid to long term. As well as monitoring service users' progress medically with their treating doctor or psychiatrist, the purpose of these interventions is also to explore connection to community and meaningful activity. Social workers are often employed as case managers. They develop individual support and recovery plans for people they work with, and lead discussions regarding treatment within the multidisciplinary team.

Community Mental Health Services

With an emphasis on psycho-social support, community mental health services are often provided by non-government, charity, and/or community grassroots organisations who noted a need. No longer seen in medical terms as an absence of symptoms, recovery is regarded as a deeply personal journey of one person's coming to terms with his or her mental illness and working towards one's own life goals. In each geographical area, these services appear differently. Potential services users need to be assessed for eligibility. For those eligible for a support package these services can then provide supports to engage in several areas such as housing, employment and activities of daily living.

Additional Settings within Mental Health Where Social Workers Are Employed

Apart from those areas already mentioned, work in interdisciplinary adult mental health practice may involve co-operating with social workers in various sectors including: aged psychiatry, youth, children; primary mental health care; and regional or state-wide services, for example forensic services and Indigenous mental health services. There are also specialist units such as eating disorders, mother-baby, extended care and personality disorders units.

Working in an Interdisciplinary Team

Multidisciplinary teams involve different health professionals working to assist the same service users. Stone (2009) refers to the term interdisciplinary team as one where there is more co-operation and communication among health professionals than the former and favours the term inter-professional collaborative team:

> This team represents a joint intellectual effort of working together in mutually supportive teams optimising the skills and knowledge of each individual to the fullest extent ... In practice this ideally translates as working towards common goals to achieve a quality experience for consumers.
>
> (Stone 2009, pp. 3, 4)

The team model varies with the setting and the social work role within it. At times, there are some challenges to overcome. These can include complexities of decision making, hierarchy, the range of knowledge and expertise and dealing with group dynamics (Renouf & Meadows, 2012). To contribute to the positive workings of the team, for the benefit of service users and families, social workers are encouraged to learn as much as they can about team practice from reading relevant literature and attending staff development. It can be useful taking a strengths-based approach to colleagues as much as service users.

What is the Role of the Social Worker?

According to the *Practice Standards for Mental Health Social Workers*:

> Social Work practice occurs at the interface between the individual and the environment: social work activity begins with the individual, and extends to the contexts of family, social networks, community, and the broader society.
>
> (Australian Association of Social Workers, 2014, p. 7)

Each social work position or generic position for which social workers are eligible to apply will have a detailed job description outlining in general terms responsibilities, key selection criteria, necessary qualifications and lines of accountability. It is advisable that social workers are familiar with the expectations of the organisation both explicit and implicit when applying for and accepting a position.

Daily Tasks of Social Workers

Daily tasks vary depending on the social work position in which employed. For example, when working in an in-patient psychiatric unit, the social work tasks are different from those completed by a social worker employed as a case manager. While there is overlap with others employed in an inpatient unit, there are tasks that the social worker alone does. Whether social workers work within a ward or case management team, there are often daily handovers outlining any incidents which occurred the day before for follow up. It is also a chance for the team to come together to discuss any pressing matters. Social workers are often called upon to support access to housing and welfare payments and are expected to have knowledge in these areas.

Specific Tasks

Often social workers begin their careers in clinical mental health working in in-patient settings. To prepare social workers for this environment, the following section outlines specific tasks expected of the in-patient social worker. Working in an Inpatient Unit is a busy, diverse, and interesting practice. It involves at least 14 distinct tasks or aspects of the role, though not all will be used with every client:

1 Meeting the person at least twice.
2 Clarifying the reason for the referral.
3 Listening.
4 Being mindful of rights.
5 Asking about significant others.
6 Linking with community agencies.
7 Supporting the person to come to terms with loss and trauma.
8 Providing psychoeducation.
9 Aiding recovery.
10 Engaging in advocacy.
11 Restricting liberties short term if it will support longer-term recovery.
12 Conducting groups
13 Participating in professional development.
14 Contributing to research.

Meeting the Person at Least Twice

The main aim of the first interview is to establish rapport. The person might still be profoundly influenced by their acute psychiatric symptoms, it might not be possible or prudent for them to make life decisions.

Clarifying the Reason for the Referral

It is important initially to clarify the reason for the referral. The person concerned may have a very different perception of their situation and need for social work involvement than the person who referred them.

Listening

Social workers are trained to be active listeners. That being the case it is important to carefully listen to the person's request using micro-skills such as being attentive to body language and where appropriate reflecting the content of what is being said and associated feelings (Geldard & Geldard, 2009).

Being Mindful of Rights

Social workers need to be equipped to provide information. Service users' rights are enshrined in the Victorian Mental Health Act 2014 and its equivalent in other states and countries. When admitted service users must be provided with information about their rights. However, it is worth checking they have understood them. Service users may require more information or linking with legal services.

Asking about Significant Others

Despite the emphasis on family sensitive practice, staff do not engage with family members as often as could be beneficial. It is vital that social workers ask about significant others and when possible arrange to meet relatives or carers with the person in the unit.

This includes asking about children, especially dependent children and meeting them too, if the person agrees it is to their benefit.

Linking with Community Agencies

The social worker can link people with other services such as counselling in a Community Health Centre so that they do not need to be part of the mental health system. For example, if someone was admitted for a situational crisis. Other examples of community agencies are Mental Health Community Support Services, housing agencies, child welfare agencies or programs at Community Health Centres such as help with gambling. Many of these agencies employ social workers who are part of multi-disciplinary or interdisciplinary teams with whom the inpatient social worker can liaise.

Supporting the Person Come to Terms with Loss and Trauma

By establishing rapport, the social worker can begin to assist the person to discuss the enormous loss and trauma that some feel after being admitted to a psychiatric institution and being diagnosed with a serious mental illness.

Providing Psychoeducation

Together with medical and nursing staff it is expected social workers provide information of a general nature to service users, carers and families. This could also involve linking to self-help organisations such as Tandem for families and carers and VIMIAC, the peak body for service users providing information and mutual support.

Aiding Recovery

Along with other staff there is the opportunity to begin discussing recovery and what this means for the person concerned and his/her family. The personal journey of recovery is now enshrined in national policy that mental health staff in all services are meant to practise (Department of Health, 2011).

Engaging in Advocacy

Advocating for service users and their families never stops whether social workers are employed in specialised or generic roles. It is important for social workers to clarify what it is they are being asked to do and how the person wants to engage (Moss, 2008, p. 27). When social workers collaborate with peer workers and lived experience advocates for service users and carers respectively, individual service users benefit greatly. At a service development level this collaboration could mean engaging in joint projects. Portfolios that staff, including social workers, undertakes such as women's rights and children of parents with mental illness are areas where advocacy is required both within and outside the organisation.

Restricting Liberties in the Short Term if it Will Support Longer-Term Recovery

In what might seem a contradiction, as well as advocating for people's rights, it might fall to the social worker to work in a way that restricts service users' liberties. An example of this is applying to the Victorian Civil Administrative Tribunal (VCAT) for an administrator when someone's illness adversely affects their managing their own finances to such a degree that they are at serious risk.

Conducting Groups

An important intervention used by social workers is groupwork; it was more common in Inpatient Units before deinstitutionalisation, however, still occurs today. Examples of group work carried out in in-patient settings involve skills development (e.g. Cooking groups); psycho-education groups (often co-facilitated with nursing staff for people to learn more about their illness); and health groups (e.g. yoga).

Participating in Professional Development

As well as attending relevant professional development within and outside the organisation social workers can be actively involved in its implementation. Examples include working with others in the team to develop a staff development program or contributing to the staff agenda for staff development from one's portfolio (e.g. parents with mental illness and their children).

Contributing to Research

Social work – with its emphasis on the person in their family and community environment, and a commitment to advocacy with and on behalf of vulnerable individuals and groups (Australian Association of Social Workers, 2010) – is a natural contributing profession to research in mental health practice. Surprisingly perhaps, however, the social work voice in this space has been a quiet one, largely utilised to support service users in raising their own voices in modest qualitative studies regarding the lived experience of health service utilisation (Hyde et al., 2014). It has been argued that social workers should engage more vocally in research:

> Indeed, the reluctance of the workforce and of employers to participate in research, to co-own it and to even understand in full its importance is one of the more central weaknesses of the profession as a whole, but one that has affected directly the power of mental health social work. This is an area in which improved collaboration between researchers, practitioners, employers, users and carers could make a difference for the future of mental health social work.
>
> (Ramon 2009, p. 1, 620)

This research could be worker-initiated research, such as the Mums' and Dads' Project, a parent education program the first author conducted and evaluated (Alakus, 2004; Alakus et al., 2007) for parents who were service users of a Melbourne Area Mental Health Service. Alternatively, the research could be part of quality improvement by a service. An example is case managers systematically recording Early Warning Signs (EWS) for all service users on their Individual Service Plans (ISP), an initiative that was piloted by an inner-city Area Mental Health Service where the first author of this chapter worked as a case manager.

Theories that Can Guide Practice

In addition to those explored in the previous chapter, there are several theories and approaches that social workers utilise in working in mental health. Some examples of tailored and targeted therapies are cognitive behavioural therapy, interpersonal therapy, supportive psychotherapy (Bland et al., 2015, p. 119), acceptance and commitment therapy and dialectical behavioural therapy. There are introductory and comprehensive courses offered to practicing social workers to develop skills in these areas.

A commitment to anti-oppressive practice (Maidment & Egan, 2004), an awareness of systems theories and problem-solving models (Coady & Lehmann, 2008) constitute important knowledge that social workers can use in their daily work. The use of interview methodologies from narrative therapy (White & Epston, 1990) works very well with clients who are being seen longer term. Feminist theories refined by practitioners such as Dominelli (2004) and Luepnitz (1988) inspire work with individuals and families as do the pioneering ideas of Hatfield and Lefley (1987) in supporting families or people with mental illness especially families from culturally and linguistically diverse backgrounds.

Reflection: Miriam's Story

Miriam was a 24-year-old single Arabic woman diagnosed with bipolar disorder who discussed her symptoms and treatments knowledgeably but never attended her appointments for depot medications punctually. Over the years her social worker and case manager made every effort to gain her trust. The ISP identified her early warning signs (EWS) and included a plan to deal with these. Her ISP included contact with family (Miriam only ever approved telephone contact) and assisting Miriam to pursue her education.

Most importantly from Miriam's point-of-view the social worker provided information and counselling about the implications of her illness for having children, something she wanted to do (see Department of Health and Ageing, Australian Infant Child Adolescent and Family Mental Health Association, 2004). With the support of a case manager, Miriam was able to avoid a serious relapse of her symptoms and a hospital admission for the first time in six years. However, Miriam was also placed on a Community Treatment Order (CTO). This was crucial in preventing relapse but was something from which Miriam wanted to eventually be liberated.

Key Practice Questions

1. Miriam's mother telephones the social worker/case manager at a time when Miriam is not present. How does the social worker engage with her mother and provide support and psycho-education while respecting Miriam's privacy?
2. When Miriam's hearing before the Mental Health Tribunal is due and the social worker arranges to be present, how does she support Miriam's wish to be self-determining recognising that the Treatment Order has ensured her treatment and extended her time out of hospital?

Reflection: Andrea's Story

Andrea was a young mother of baby, Lucas. Her partner and the baby's father was Steven. Andrea's diagnosis was schizoaffective disorder and severe anxiety complicated by alcohol dependence. Case management included working with Andrea in her new role as a parent, involving her and her partner in psycho-education and discussing community resources for new parents and babies. The baby became an active participant in sessions providing an opportunity to praise Andrea and her partner on the great job they were doing as parents.

As one of Andrea's prime goals was to get help with her anxiety, she also saw a psychologist at the service for cognitive behavioural therapy. The anxiety was linked to Andrea's battle with alcohol that surfaced as the main problem from time to time. Help could be sought from the drug and alcohol team based at the service when Andrea was ready.

Andrea's partner proved a responsible parent and supported Andrea but made it clear there was a limit to how much he would tolerate her abuse of alcohol. All the while the social worker as case manager, who had gained Andrea's trust by supporting her through her pregnancy, continued to monitor her mental health with the treating doctor. Equally important was monitoring Lucas's safety. At that point his physical and emotional needs were being met and there was another adult in his life who could attend to these needs should Andrea's condition relapse.

A long term goal in her ISP was to resume her career as a singing teacher.

Key Practice Questions

1 At what point does the social worker consult or involve drug and alcohol services?
2 When might it be necessary to involve child and family services?

The Strengths of Mental Health Social Workers

Social workers are a useful asset to clinical mental health teams. They bring different perspectives to multidisciplinary teams, often raising ideas which are not traditionally considered by medical professions. Social workers often consider alternate explanation for symptoms that require social interventions (rather than medication changes). Reflecting on a person's environment; their history; their current stressors as well as symptoms experienced can provide a broader explanation of their presentation. Having a trauma-informed approach, social workers are able to support organisations be more appropriate in their language and processes that create trauma informed workplaces. Social workers have a strong commitment to social justice (Australian Association of Social Workers, 2010), which is integral in ensuring service users have access to support which is not going to further traumatise them. Social workers value the lived experience of service users and their families (Bland et al., 2015, p. 119) advocating on their behalf at all levels of care. Social workers have a strong dedication to addressing disadvantage, a core aspect of practice, and ideologically oppose poverty and other social experiences which impact on service users. Social workers recognise the marginalisation of those who experience mental health issues, including the stigma faced, and actively work to counter-act this. In Australia, Social workers are also able to become accredited mental health social workers (by the Australian Association of Social Workers after meeting several practice and academic obligations). Once accredited, private social work sessions are able to be subsidised under Medicare (a national publicly funded health care scheme). Social workers are integral to mental health services, and continue to grow and contribute to all areas of mental health service delivery.

Surviving and Thriving

Social work in mental health requires dedication and stamina. To continue to be effective several strategies can be helpful. One strength of social work is the capacity to critically reflect. *Critical reflection* is defined as 'a process that fosters integration of self, theory and practice in a way that is dynamic, sharpening our view and understanding of factors that influence the way we think and behave towards others' (Maidment & Egan, 2004, p. 14). This can be done individually, for instance by keeping a journal and/or enhanced in supervision. This is helpful in and of itself, but also helps prepare for supervision.

Social work *supervision* is of such importance that it is mentioned in the Practice Standards for Mental Health Social Workers (Australian Association of Social Workers, 2014, p. 25). If for some reason supervision is not available or adequate within the organisation, it is worth arranging for it externally. Alongside formal supervision, *support* from other social workers from within the service or elsewhere is important. Meeting regularly with social work colleagues for work related matters also informally helps maintains a social work identity.

Many opportunities exist in mental health services for *staff development*, both within organisations and through others such as Mental Health Victoria. Online opportunities are also available such as MHPOD. A professional person also *reads*; this should be something that continues after graduation. In the case of social workers in mental health it includes material on mental health, policy changes, social work textbooks, journal articles and website information of organisations that assist people with a mental illness, their families and carers. Over time *extra study*, such as a higher degree in social work or family therapy, can be a useful way of learning new ideas and sustaining interest.

Joining your professional body – in Australia the Australian Association of Social Workers (AASW) – is recommended since it is a good source of information, support and action. The AASW Code of Ethics is available from the AASW website and is worth consulting regularly. It is important too for social work practitioners to *work out priorities*. It is simply not possible to do everything at once. New graduates may focus mostly on case work and learning. With progress in the field they may take on policy or an advocacy role. With time social workers can be more confident of achieving more of the changes they have been working towards. Self-care is vital so it is important that social workers remember that they are human beings too. While they generally encourage it for service users, it is important that social workers *take regular time out* to enjoy life, exercise and care for their own health.

If Experiences Are Causing Distress

After trying all the items suggested under surviving and thriving, if things are still not working out, it may be time to consider a change of job. Big organisations offer opportunities in other parts of the service. Another possibility is to transfer to another area of social work because the experience in one area can greatly enhance a social worker's contribution in another. Alternatively one can do something completely different for a while and return invigorated.

Conclusion

It is an exciting time to be a social worker in mental health. Preceding decades have seen radical changes in resources and care being transferred from big isolated psychiatric hospitals to Area Mental Health Services. That the reforms may not have gone far enough is due in part to a society that does not pay sufficient attention to social determinants of health such as employment, income security, housing and education. Whatever their involvement, whether it be as a case manager or working in an inpatient unit, for example social workers need to be aware of societal changes and contribute where possible to policy debate and research both individually and collectively. In doing so, it is crucial social workers collaborate with service users and carers.

Key Website Resources

Bouverie Centre (www.bouverie.org.au). Provides clinical family therapy and community education.

Children of Parents with a Mental Illness (www.copmi.net.au). Includes many resources useful for parents, children, family, friends and helping professionals.

MHPOD (www2.health.voc.gov.au). An evidence-based online learning resource for staff working in mental health including social workers.

Mental Health Victoria (www.mhvic.org.au). The peak body for the community managed service sector.

Tandem (www.tandemcarers.org.au). The peak body for families and carers of people with mental illness in Victoria.

References

Alakus, C. (2004). Learning together about the needs of parents with a mental illness and their children: The implementation of the Mums' and Dads' Practice Research Project. *Children Australia*, 29(2), 35–40.

Alakus, C., Conwell, R., Gilbert, M., Buist, A. & Castle, D. (2007). The needs of parents with a mental illness who have young children: An Australian perspective on service delivery options. *International Journal of Social Psychiatry*, 53(4), 333–339.

Australian Association of Social Workers. (2010). *Code of Ethics*. Australian Association of Social Workers.

Australian Association of Social Workers. (2014). *The Practice Standards for Mental Health Social Workers*. Australian Association of Social Workers.

Bland, R. (2012). The social worker. In G. Meadows *et al., Mental Health in Australia Collaborative Community Practice* (pp. 290–294). New York: Oxford University Press.

Bland, R., Renouf, N. and Tullgren, A. (2015) *Social Work Practice in Mental Health: An Introduction*. Sydney: Allen & Unwin.

Chenoweth, L. & McAuliffe, D. (2005) *The Road to Social Work & Human Service Practice*. South Melbourne: Thomson.

Coady, N. & Lehmann, P. (2008) *Theoretical Perspectives for Direct Social Work Practice A Generalist-Eclectic Approach*, 2nd edition. New York: Springer.

Department of Health and Ageing, Australian Infant Child Adolescent and Family Mental Health Association. (2004). *The Best for Me and My Baby*. Department of Health and Ageing, Australian Infant Child Adolescent and Family Mental Health Association.

Department of Health. (2011) *Framework for Recovery-Oriented Practice*. State Government of Victoria.

Dominelli, L. (2004). *Social Work: Theory and Practice for a Changing Profession*. Cambridge: Cambridge University Press.

Geldard, D. & Geldard, K. (2009) *Basic Personal Counselling*, 7th edition. Frenchs Forest, NSW: Pearson.

Hatfield, A. B. & Lefley, H. P. (eds). (1987). *Families of Mentally Ill: Coping and Adaptation*. New York: Guilford Press.

Human Services Victoria Mental Health Branch (1994). *Victoria's Mental Health Services: The Framework for Service Delivery*:Melbourne: Human Services Victoria Mental Health Branch.

Hyde, B., Bowles, W. & Pawar, M. (2014). Challenges of recovery-oriented practice in inpatient mental health settings: The potential for social work leadership. *Asia Pacific Journal of Social Work and Development*, 24(1–2), 5–16.

Leggatt, M. & Jeffs, S. (2020). *Out of the Madhouse: From Asylums to Caring Community?*Acadia.

Luepnitz, D. A. (1988). *The Family Interpreted, Psychoanalysis, Feminism and Family Therapy*. New York: Basic Books.

Maidment, J. & Egan, R. (eds). (2004). *Practice Skills in Social Work & Welfare More than just common sense*. Crows Nest, NSW: Allen & Unwin.

Moss, B. (2008). *Communication skills for health and social care*. London: Sage.

Papakotsias, A. & Zimmerman, A. (2012). *Housing and Support: A decent place to live and call home*. In G. Meadow et al. (eds), *Mental Health in Australia: Collaborative Community Practice* (p. 506). Oxford: Oxford University Press.

Ramon, S. (2009). Adult mental health in a changing international context: The relevance to social work. *British Journal of Social Work*, 39(8), 1615–1622.

Renouf, N. & Meadows, G. (2012). *Working collaboratively in teams*. In G. Meadow et al. (eds), *Mental Health in Australia: Collaborative Community Practice* (pp. 301–306). Oxford: Oxford University Press.

Rosen, A. (2006). The Australian experience of deinstitutionalization: Interaction of Australian culture with the development and reform of its mental health services. *Acta Psychiatrica Scandinavica*, 113 (s429), 81–89.

Saxena, S., Kane, J., Krawczyk, N. & Bass, J. K. (2019). *Mental Health Systems Around the World*. New York: Oxford University Press.

Shen, G. C., Snowden, L. R. (2014). Institutionalization of deinstitutionalization: A cross-national analysis of mental health system reform. *International Journal of Mental Health Systems*, 8, 47.

Stone, J. (2009). *International Collaborative Practice (PCP): Definitions and Terminology*. ACT Health.

White, M. & Epston, D. (1990). *Narrative Means to Therapeutic Ends*. New York: W. W. Norton.

Austin, W. (2017). Global health ethics and mental health. In E. Yearwood & V. Hines-Martin (eds), *Routledge Handbook of Global Mental Health Nursing* (pp. 93–112). New York: Routledge.

8 Aged Care

Health, Assessments, In-Home Care and Residential Care

Lisa Braddy, Mara Erhardt-Rumpe and Penny Lording

Older people constitute a highly diverse group. Many lead active and healthy lives while some much younger 'older people' have poorer quality of life (World Health Organization, 2021). Each person's experience of ageing is unique and influenced by a variety of factors including genetics, physical and social environments and personal characteristics including; gender, ethnicity, family size, life skills, migration history and work experience (World Health Organization, 2021). Although many older people experience a number of health conditions, intrinsic capacity to function in their environment is a better predictor of health and well-being than the absence of disease.

Expertise in managing the complex, multi-faceted issues in aged care is a requirement of social workers in health-based positions. Aged care lies at the interface of Australia's health and social welfare systems. Social workers navigate an important role in ensuring the rights of the older person are upheld while facilitating their continued independence and well-being in the context of their changing health needs.

The Australian population is living longer. Australia has one of the highest life expectancies in the world, at 82.8 years in 2018 for males and females at birth combined – ranked seventh among 37 Organisation for Economic Co-operation and Development (OECD) countries. There have also been increases in the expected number of healthy years (World Health Organization, 2016). In 2017, 15% of Australia's total population were aged 65 and over, that is 1 in 7 people; by 2057 it is projected that those aged 65 years and over will make up 22% of the Australian population (Australian Institute of Health and Welfare, 2021).

An analysis of Australian Health Survey data indicates consultation with health professionals and health care services increases with age. Around 20% of people over the age of 65 are admitted to hospital compared with 11% of people under 65 (Australian Institute of Health and Welfare, 2014). Older people represent a significant proportion of the cohort that health Social Workers interact with and support. As demand increases, the associated financial pressures impact on patient throughput in hospitals and increasing the reliance on community-based service delivery (Nilsson & Braddy, 2009). This has led to many hospitals delivering home-based Geriatric Evaluation and Management (GEM) admissions (Northern Health, 2021; Eastern Health, 2021).

The interrelationship between social structures and complex health care creates challenges for the health and aged care systems. Flexibility in the range of services available, how they are delivered and funding models will need to change.

Major issues confronting the Australian health care system in the next decade include:

DOI: 10.4324/9781003330745-10

- Increasing rates of chronic illness.
- Demand for health and aged care services increasing at a faster rate than funding for additional capacity.
- Increased individual spending on health care and increased consumer expectations of timely access to and quality of service.
- Need for different models of care and workforce practices to utilise a wider range of treatment possibilities and new technologies in response to demand.
- A predicted move of older people to the outer suburbs or regional areas and at greater distances from families than previous generations.
- Alterations in policy delivery and service development to reflect the diversity of older Australians.
- Increased average age of health workers in a landscape where health workforce supply already fails to keep up with demand.(Macri, 2016)

Current Sector Reform

Health Reform

National health care priorities change in response to shifts in demographics, social and economic conditions and emerging technology. This includes a significant increase in the use of telehealth to address barriers to care provision as a result of the COVID-19 pandemic, although not all groups have access to or knowledge of the technology required to utilise these options (Fisk, Livingstone & Pit, 2020). Total spending on health in 2019–2020 is estimated to be $81.8 billion, representing 16.3 per cent of the Australian Government's total expenditure (Parliamentary Library, 2021).

Since the 1990s, health service delivery was focused on efficiency and outputs via a funding model known as 'case-mix funding'. This involved a shift to a nationally consistent approach to funding health services based on multiple factors related to the patient, their main diagnosis on admission and any medically or socially complicating factors. 'The Travis Review' (2015) represents a further major shift. The recommendations from this review aimed at increasing capacity in Victorian hospitals and delivering better patient outcomes focused on: patient experience, access, adverse events, prevention and cost. It highlighted the importance of building capacity through innovation and not new buildings (Travis, 2015). In addition, there has been an increased focus on ensuring that care is delivered in a safe way without causing avoidable harm to patients (Duckett, Cuddihy & Newnham, 2016).

A challenge for social workers is to ensure that clinical services are delivered and redesigned for maximum efficiency while maintaining quality of care across the continuum (Nicol, Mohanna & Cowpe, 2014). Social workers have an important role in improving quality of care, patient safety and the organisation's performance.

Aged Care Reform

There have been a number of major reforms of the aged care sector in Australia. These have broadly encompassed the following themes: a greater emphasis on choice and control for the older person; a continued emphasis on a user pays system, with co-payments and means-tested fees and an increasing prioritisation of enablement and wellness approaches with the older person as an active agent in maintaining their independence.

To support these objectives, the provision of additional in-home support services to maintain an older person's independence, increased choice and improved access to a range of health and aged care services have been introduced. Increased support introduced for informal carers and family, acknowledge the important role they play in maintaining an older person's health and independence; with enhanced access to information about aged care services through a centralised resource, increased monitoring of quality and safety of residential aged care services and pricing transparency, as well as carer support services.

These reforms are a direct response to the Royal Commission into Aged Care Quality and Safety, which was established in 2018 and delivered their Final Report in early 2021. Recommendations were underpinned by a strong rights-based approach.

Reform to Community-Based Aged Care Provision

Providing quality care is more than simply meeting basic needs. Changing demography and social norms challenge the capacity of families to meet the care needs of a dependent older person alone. Responsibility for long-term care is ideally shared between families, governments and other sectors in order to safeguard access to quality care (World Health Organization, 2016).

In 2018–2019 1.1% of GDP was spent on aged care by the Australian government. The aged care system offers two mainstream care options for older people: community-based and residential aged care. Commonly, people enter the aged care system through community-based care and if needed progress to residential care. In 2017–2018, 7% of Australians 65 years and over accessed residential aged care while an additional 22% received home care (Australian Government, 2016). Of note, in 2017–2018, 71% of Australians aged 65 and over lived at home without accessing government funded aged care services. To better support the principles of aged care discussed there has been an overall shift from funding residential care to increased funding of community-based care.

The My Aged Care Gateway became operational from July 2015. It aims to streamline access to the aged care system and simplify pathways for older people through levels of care as their needs change. My Aged Care functions as a central point of access for information, assessment and referral to Commonwealth funded aged care services. The gateway also facilitates: a central client record accessed by a web-based portal; a standardised approach to screening and assessments of older people seeking access to aged care services; and electronic referrals for assessment and/or services.

Accessed via My Aged Care, the Commonwealth Home Support Programme (CHSP) provides entry-level services focused on supporting older people to maintain their independence in the community. Home Care Packages build on informal networks providing access to tailored supports and case management. A consumer directed approach underpins delivery and encourages the older person to choose their service provider.

Residential care in Australia is Commonwealth funded and offered by both not-for-profit and private providers. It is intended to support older people whose health needs can no longer be met by community-based services. Social workers assist older people and their carers to navigate the aged care system, to facilitate access to those services and to provide support throughout the process. This is often a confusing and stressful time for the older person, as frequently the need for more formal support has been prompted by increasing health issues and complex psycho-social factors.

Consumer Directed Care

The disability and aged care sectors continue to experience significant systems transition and reform. In 2010 Consumer Directed Care (CDC) was introduced across all Commonwealth funded Home Care Packages. This approach emphasises greater choice and control for the older person and enhanced flexibility. Under a CDC approach, older people are supported to identify goals within the context of independence, wellness and re-ablement. The consumer controls the level of involvement they want in managing their package, the types of support services they wish to access and who delivers these. Through an individualised budget, CDC provides greater transparency to the consumer about funding that is available. This has challenged traditional models of case management which has a strong social work workforce. The case manager role has a greater focus on facilitating well-being and an advisory role – 'doing with' rather than 'doing for'. The challenges faced by people in accessing and co-ordinating their care requires a strengthened involvement of social workers as advocates and coaches is crucial (McCallum & Rees, 2017).

Role of Social Work in Health

Social work practice in health environments has a long tradition reaching back to the origins of the profession in the late nineteenth and early twentieth centuries. Training of hospital social workers in Australia commenced in Sydney and Melbourne in the late 1920s. Hospital social work practice has developed in response to evolving health care contexts such as changes in disease patterns, treatment and service redesign (Nilsson & Braddy, 2009).

At an organisational level social workers contribute to equitable access to health care and identify system barriers that potentially affect the older person's engagement and participation in their care. A social worker's skillset contributes to promoting the older person's voice in the development of culturally appropriate and person-centred service responses. Social workers utilise their expertise to prevent hospital readmissions and reduce inappropriate health service use by rigorous discharge planning, risk assessment and addressing psychosocial factors in their interventions (Australian Association of Social Workers, 2020). As a health professional they undertake an active role in evidence-based service redesign and evaluation to ensure that clinical interventions are delivered efficiently while maintaining quality of care (Nicol, Mohanna & Cowpe, 2014).

Hospital social work plays a pivotal role in addressing psychosocial issues resulting from illness, disability and hospitalisation (Cleak & Turczynski, 2014). This is undertaken using a range of interventions including: psychosocial screening and assessment, identification of risk, safety planning, counselling, impact and adjustment to illness, advocacy, internal and external referral, information, education and provision of resource entitlements. With an ageing population social work in a health context considers the needs of the older person focussing on family networks and connections, community support and engagement, legal and financial issues, access to community packages of care, adjustment to chronic illness, residential aged care, disability services, family violence and neglect (Nilsson & Braddy, 2009).

Health social workers assess the older person in the context of their usual environment. This bio-psycho-social approach enables them to be considered in the context of their lived experience, beyond the narrow limits of their illness or disability through the lens of the social determinants of health. Such an approach aids in identifying what supports may be available or needed upon discharge. Hospitals are highly professional work environments and social workers need to operate effectively within a medical model of service delivery. Written communication is formal in style. Assessment is a fundamental tool of the social worker which is used to highlight psycho-social barriers to timely discharge, but is ineffective without highly developed written and verbal skills to communicate the patient's story (Nilsson & Braddy, 2009).

Role of Social Work in Community Aged Care

Social workers are employed in a variety of roles in the community and residential aged care sectors. Some roles are social work specific; others are generic, e.g. assessment officers and case managers.

The main focus of intervention is maintaining the older person's level of independence, provide monitoring, and enhance well-being, facilitate connection to community, and the provision of practical and emotional support. Often this means that social workers are involved with older people over a lengthy period, particularly if they hold a case management role. These professionals are an important source of information about the older person's pre-morbid functioning and well-being, which can be drawn upon if the person is admitted to hospital. In this context, community based social workers will generally resume responsibility for the continuum of care once the older person is discharged from hospital.

Theoretical frameworks

In addition to the bio-psycho-social approach, social work practice in health and community aged care is underpinned and informed by the following frameworks and theories:

- Strengths based practice – to ensure the older person's abilities and experiences are utilised and reinforce strengths and previous coping capacities in times of deteriorating health and changing needs.
- Family centred practice – to ensure family roles and dynamics are considered in the context of the older person's life, and recognising the role that family plays in the provision of support.
- Narrative therapy – often used as a tool to gain a holistic picture of the older person and to identify their strengths and what is important to them.
- Social role valorisation – a framework that facilitates the older person's ongoing contribution to their local community despite the impact of changing health and increasing frailty.
- Trauma informed approach – is based on the understanding that trauma can be cumulative and impact the person, their emotions and relationships with others over the course of their lifetime. Core practice principles include safety, trust, choice, collaboration, empowerment and respect for diversity.
- Brief intervention – is particularly relevant to a hospital setting where a person may be admitted for a short time resulting in the Social Worker needing to adopt a more solution or task focussed approach. This ensures that the concerns most relevant to the person can be addressed and a plan developed for longer term concerns to be followed up in the community.

- Evidence informed practice – in health care and aged care, there is an increasing use of validated assessment tools which the beginning practitioner needs to become familiar with as part of an evidence informed approach to practice. It is also important to maintain knowledge of the latest research to inform social work practice.
- Coaching – An approach which acknowledges the older person as the expert in their own lives and the role of the practitioner is one of facilitator and advisor.
- Goal setting – a collaborative approach on that encourages the older person with changing health needs to identify what is most important to them in terms of quality of life and then working together to determine the types of supports which will enable the achievement of these goals.
- Co-design and co-production – more recently co-design methodologies and approaches have been seen in community aged care, with a focus on ensuring older people are equal partners in service planning, delivery, governance and evaluation.

Issues to Consider When Working with Older People

Dignity of Risk vs Duty of Care

Disability and old age do not equate incapacity to make decisions. Older people *do not* give up their right to make decisions or actively participate in the process during hospitalisation or while accessing community support services, unless there is a formal medical diagnosis and assessment of mental capacity that determines they are unable to make some or all decisions for themselves.

When working with older people it is important that social workers have an understanding of capacity, competency, dementia and effects of cognitive changes on the ability to make informed decisions. A person with capacity is free to reject reasonable and appropriate recommendations. The older person may decline the recommendations put forward by a health professional and make different decisions to those suggested by the treating team. It is important to respect that the older person is the expert in their life and explore their preferences and identify their expectations regarding care and discharge plans.

Social workers in aged care undertake an important role in upholding the older person's right to make decisions and maintaining a focus on 'will and preference'. This ensures that older people continue to influence what happens to them, even if they are assessed as lacking capacity to make some or all decisions for themselves (Office of the Public Advocate, Victoria, 2020).

Social workers have a key role in the provision of information to facilitate informed decision making in relation to future planning. This may include arrangements such as appointing enduring powers of attorney. Social workers should also intervene appropriately where it is clear that the older person can no longer make informed decisions. Working with older people in these circumstances requires sensitivity and a well-developed understanding of relevant legislation so that the older person's rights are only impinged once less restrictive options have been attempted.

Disease Trajectory

Social workers in health and aged care generally work with older people experiencing multiple co-morbidities. It is important to understand the trajectory of diseases that commonly affect older people, including dementia, Parkinson's disease, cancer, cardiovascular disease, diabetes, arthritis, and glaucoma. This knowledge facilitates future planning with the older person and early identification of risk factors in the context of maintaining the older person's independence at home or facilitating a discharge home or to residential aged care from hospital.

Family Violence across the Lifespan

Family violence is a major public health issue. Healthcare workers have a role to play in responding to family violence and the associated health impacts (Victorian Government, 2016). The Royal Commission into Family Violence Report (2016) made 227 recommendations directed at improving the foundations of the current system and the way in which all service sectors respond to family violence.

Older people can be subject to family members who use violence with an estimated 2 to 10 per cent of older Australians experiencing abuse. Elder abuse is a relatively 'hidden' problem but as part of the assessment process, health and aged care social workers need to be aware of the risk factors for abuse and signs that indicate the older person is potentially experiencing family violence. Recent reforms in family violence legislation related to risk assessment and information sharing have helped to clarify and strengthen the role of hospital social workers in this area.

Mental Health

Depression in older people is an important public health issue, as it is associated with increased risk of morbidity and suicide, decreased cognitive, physical and social functioning, and greater self-neglect (Fiske, Loebach Wetherall & Gatz, 2009). It is thought that 10–15% of older people experience depression and about 10% experience anxiety. Rates of depression among older people living in residential aged care are thought to be much higher, around 35%. Given the high prevalence of poor mental health in the older age group, it is essential for bio-psycho-social assessments completed by hospital social workers to include a consideration of the person's mental health. Good mental health is linked with healthy ageing, therefore if indicated, it is important that social workers follow-up specialised mental health support for older people in a timely manner (Beyond Blue, 2009).

Assessment

Older people often present to hospital with non-specific symptoms. These can mask issues that occur with ageing, presenting a challenge for clinicians to identify how the older person usually lives their life. While everyone ages in a different way, ageing is generally accompanied by a decline in many homeostatic and metabolic processes. As a result assessment for older people differs to that for younger people (Victorian Government Health Hub, 2016).

It is vital to view the assessment as a 'live' and ongoing process. As Sansoni et al. (2012) highlight, assessment in aged care as a continuous, multi-tiered and multi-staged process. It informs the care pathway to services and contributes to decisions about eligibility for different levels of care. For social workers the main purpose of assessment is to:

- Identify the person's psychosocial situation – 'the person in their environment'.
- Purposefully gather information to aid in improved outcomes – such as enhanced quality of life and reduced carer burden. Many older people's problems go

unreported, undetected and untreated. It important for the social worker to adopt an approach of 'curious enquiry' when completing an assessment.
- Build a collaborative relationship with the older person and where relevant, their family and other sources of significant formal or informal support.
- Develop an intervention plan based on contracting and goal setting to inform implementation.

The hospital treating team often focuses on an older person's acute health problems but social workers take a broader perspective that includes the person's psychosocial needs which can impact on outcomes. While social work assessments in hospital and community settings, identify risks to the older person's independence, there is also increasingly a focus on well-being and goals which enable the older person to live their life the way they choose. Developing a person-centred plan that actively engages the older person is an integral part of effective care planning (Victorian Government Health Hub, 2016). The 'Psychosocial Assessment Domains' box presents domains that are considered by social workers when completing psychosocial assessments.

Psychosocial Assessment Domains

Introduction

Source of and reason for referral
Key points from hospital progress entries – *admissions, diagnoses, investigations, team input, events, planning*
Source(s) of information

Living Situation

Current accommodation – *type, ownership, location, access, timeframe*
Household composition. How the person identifies and interfaces with their community
Protective or risk factors identified
Potential barriers to care or discharge

Lifestyle and Activities of Daily Living (ADIs)

Usual ADLs – *personal, domestic, community*
Level of independence with ADLs, mobility
Aids and equipment used
Physical, cognitive, mental health issues impacting on function
Employment, education, interests, social engagement, substance/alcohol use (if relevant) or other issues that impact equitable access on the care pathway

Informal/Family Supports

Person's relationship status and preferred pronouns
How the person interfaces, identifies and connects with their community
Indigenous/Non Indigenous
Primary carer and next of kin details
Family structure/family members' input – *contact, involvement, relationship*
Culture, ethnicity, migration history (if relevant)

Formal Supports

Community services – *type, organisation, frequency, timeframe*
Case management – *organisation, contact person and details, timeframe*
Other/specialist services involved

Financial/Legal Situation

Income – *type, source, adequacy, timeframe*
Ability to manage finances/persons involved or assisting
Legal instruments, e.g. Enduring Power of Attorney, Guardianship – *type, persons involved, contact details*

Adjustment to Illness

Attitude to hospitalisation and treatment – *insight, concerns, coping, immediate wellbeing, expectations*
Current emotional state – *reported, observed by Social Worker*
Prior experience of illness – *coping strategies, supports, strengths, concerns*
Family adjustment – *insight, concerns, coping, expectations*

Cognition

Confusion or altered state – *degree, duration, history, key events, impact on functioning*

Carer Issues

Carer's situation – *physical and mental wellbeing, concerns, supports, needs, capacity to continue care*

Expectations Regarding Discharge (if in Hospital)

Discharge date/timeframe – *insight, hopes, patient and family expectations*
Discharge destination – *location, supports, issues, barriers*

Outcome/Implications

Summary and prioritisation of identified psychosocial issues
Current care management issues – *medical, nursing, allied health, other*
Potential risks, suspected abuse or conflict of interest – *current management, discharge planning*
Person/family acceptance or otherwise of situation and treating team plan

Action/Intervention

Steps taken to address identified issues – *liaison, discussion, meetings, care and safety planning, referrals, counselling*

Plan

Outstanding tasks required to address identified issues – *by Social Worker, team, person, family*

Anticipated timeframes and outcomes
Social Work position re proposed care or discharge plan – *agreement, disagreement, suggestions*

In individualising the assessment, social workers tailor their report to reflect the current presentation and communicate their professional opinion to the target audience. Case notes in health records provide evidence of critical thinking, clinical reasoning and the decision making process when providing care. All documentation should be relevant to the presenting issues and be factual and succinct.

A focus on responding to potential system barriers and equity issues can strengthen the older person's experience of care. Dilemmas of privacy and confidentiality can arise and social workers should be mindful that the medical record and case notes are legal documents that cannot be changed once written (Nilsson & Braddy, 2009). Additionally, under Freedom of Information the patient can access their medical record. Hence, clinical entries should be factual and clear in the professional's assessment of the situation.

Reflection: Mrs Caklais's Story

Providing optimal care for older people rarely involves a single intervention. However, the complexity of integrating multiple assessments, managing best practice interventions for different risks and integrating the older person's preferences is not a straightforward task (Victorian Government Health Hub, 2016).

The following practice exemplar has a sub-acute focus but the themes, skills and knowledge are transferrable to other settings. The example below provides details of documentation including an initial assessment and a Victorian Civil and Administrative Tribunal (VCAT) report. Other Social Work interventions in this scenario are likely to include convening a family meeting, documenting family meeting minutes, service referrals and other legal, financial or supporting letters.

Sample Initial Assessment
Social Worker
Name: Alex Jackson (pronouns: *he/they*)
Unit: Geriatric Evaluation and Management (GEM) Unit
Hospital: St Oliver's Hospital Melbourne

Patient Profile
Name: Mrs Louise Dana Caklais (pronouns: *she/her*)
Date of Admission:
Acute: 15/9/2020
Sub-acute: 16/10/2020
Address: 10 Benjamin St
Preston Vic 3072
Phone: 8342 8749
DOB: 20 August 1932 (88 years)
Country of origin: Latvia
Interpreter: Conversational English. Interpreter recommended for complex contact such as initial assessment and family meetings.
Gender: Female

Medical History

Recent history of falls resulting in fractured neck of femur
Recent history of cognitive changes and short-term memory loss
Disorientation and confusion
Past medical history includes: hypertension, diabetes, glaucoma, age-related hearing loss

Genogram

[see Figure 8.1]

Social Profile

Mrs Caklais is a widow of 20 years who lives alone in the family home. She has four children: John (63) who lives in Collingwood, Isabella (61) who lives in Fitzroy, Dana (60) who lives in Kew and Michael (58) who lives in West Preston. Children and extended family maintain daily contact and provide support as required. Mrs Caklais migrated to Australia from Latvia in 1950. She has social links with the local Latvian community. Mrs Caklais would benefit from the use of an interpreter in discussing complex decisions although she has conversational English. Mrs Caklais engaged readily with the writer.

Accommodation

Mrs Caklais resides alone in her own, single storey, home.

Legal and Financial

Recipient of partial Age pension and rental income from a second property. Previously managed own finances with informal support from Dana. Both Mrs Caklais and Dana have advised that Mrs Caklais wants to sell her second property as continuing to manage the needs of that property in relation to keeping it rented out (even with support from Dana) is now causing her some stress. No Enduring Powers of Attorney or Advanced Care Directive completed.

Transport

Community access with support of family. Has half price taxi card.

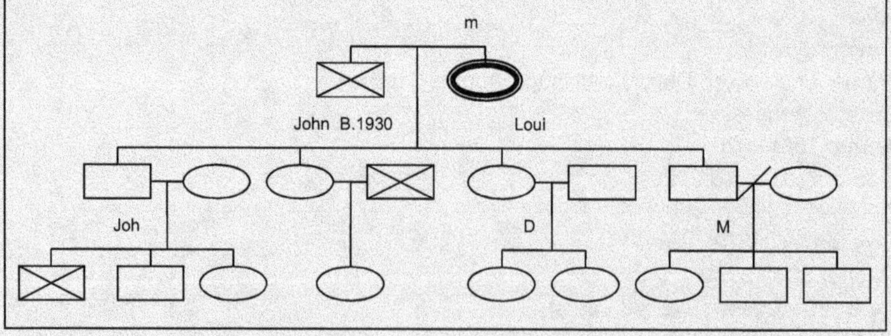

Figure 8.1 Genogram: Mrs Caklais

Formal Supports

No formal supports accessed prior to admission. Mrs Caklais' children and grandchildren provide practical assistance as required and support her with community access. Domestic tasks and meal preparation managed by Mrs Caklais' daughters. Family state they are able to continue this level of support.

ADLs

Mrs Caklais requires minimal assistance and prompting with personal care once set up. Mrs Caklais has a history of three recent falls and ambulates short distances with a single point stick. She is independent with bed mobility and transfers. Mrs Caklais is continent. She requires assistance with medication management due to impaired vision.

Cognition

Mrs Caklais is orientated to time and place but has recently experienced cognitive changes and periods of confusion. Family members have expressed concern regarding Mrs Caklais' increasing forgetfulness over the past six months. Social Work notes Occupational Therapist assessment reporting difficulty with planning and sequencing of tasks. Further cognitive assessment by Neuro-psychologist noted confirming Mrs Caklais is experiencing difficulty with complex decision making.

Expectations

Mrs Caklais highly values her independence and expressed a wish to return home post discharge. She feels that the support provided by her family is sufficient and does not wish to have any formal supports.

Sample VCAT Letter

Victorian Civil and Administrative Tribunal
Human Rights Division
Level 5 William Cooper Justice Centre
Guardianship List
Submitted via: Guardianship Hub
23 October 2020
To whom it may concern,
RE Mrs Louise Caklais (pronouns: *she/her*)
10 Benjamin Street
Preston Vic 3072
D.O.B. 20/08/1932

Introduction

It is in my capacity as Social Worker at St Oliver's Hospital that I submit the following application and request your consideration of the appointment of an Administrator for the above-mentioned patient. A neuropsychology report supporting this application is attached.

Admission Summary

Mrs Caklais was admitted to hospital following a fall at home on 15/09/2020 which resulted in a fractured neck of femur. She was transferred to the Geriatric Evaluation and Management (GEM) Unit on 16/10/2020 where she remains an inpatient. She has a recent diagnosis of dementia. Other relevant medical history includes hypertension, diabetes, glaucoma and age related hearing loss. For additional information please refer to the attached medical report.

Social Situation

Mrs Caklais is an 84 year old female of Latvian origin. A widow of 16 years she usually resides in the family home alone. She migrated to Australia in 1950 and worked as a nurse until her retirement. Prior to this hospital admission Mrs Caklais required minimal assistance with activities of daily living and support with community access. She did not access any formal supports. Mrs Caklais has four adult children who live nearby, maintain daily contact and provide practical and emotional support as required.

Finances/Legal Situation

Mrs Caklais receives a partial Age pension and rental income from a second property. She was previously supported on an informal basis to manage her own finances by her daughter, Dana. Mrs Caklais now wants to sell her second property as continuing to manage the needs of that property in relation to keeping it rented out (even with support from Dana) is now causing her significant stress. Mrs Caklais has been assessed as unable to complete more complex decision making or appoint an enduring power of attorney.

Current Function and Care Planning

Functionally Mrs Caklais ambulates short distances with a single point stick. She has poor endurance and remains at risk of falls. Mrs Caklais is independent with transfers and bed mobility. She is continent and requires minimal assistance with showering, dressing and grooming. Mrs Caklais requires prompting and supervision with administration of her medication. As noted above, she has a recent diagnosis of dementia and communicates more confidently in Latvian.

Least Restrictive Options Explored

In order to support Mrs Caklais to make financial decisions, the appointment of an Enduring Power of Attorney (Financial) was explored. Due to her level of cognitive impairment, however, Mrs Caklais has been assessed as unable to make this appointment. The option of Dana continuing to manage Mrs Caklais' finances informally was also explored, however, given the need for property to be sold, this will not be sufficient.

Matters for VCAT to Determine

It is the assessment of the GEM treating team Mrs Caklais would benefit from the appointment of an Administrator to assist her in the management of her financial affairs. Mrs Caklais has expressed her will and preference to have her daughter, Dana to continue to support her in this way. Dana is willing to take on this role and Mrs Caklais' family are supportive of this. It is considered that the appointment of an administrator will support Mrs Caklais' personal and social wellbeing by ensuring that she someone who is able to make legal and financial decisions in consultation with her.

It is requested that Mrs Caklais have access to a Latvian interpreter throughout the proceedings. She would also benefit from a hearing loop.
If you require further information, please do not hesitate to contact me on 9999 5555.
Yours sincerely
Alex Smith (pronouns: *he/they*)
Social Worker
Geriatric Evaluation and Management Unit
St Oliver's Hospital

Conclusion

Working with older people in health contexts is both a rewarding and challenging experience. It is one where the older person and the Social Worker can learn from each other and where thorough assessment, interventions and care planning can have a significant impact on the older person's quality of life.

Key Website Resources

The Global Strategy and Action Plan on Ageing and Health 2016–2020: towards a world in which everyone can live a long and healthy life:

- www.who.int/health-topics/ageing#tab=tab_1
- www.who.int/news-room/fact-sheets/detail/ageing-and-health

Community-based care provision:

- www.health.gov.au/health-topics/aged-care/aged-care-resources
- www.aph.gov.au/About_Parliament/Parliamentary_Departments/Parliamentary_Library/pubs/rp/rp1617/Quick_Guides/Aged_Care_a_quick_guide
- www.myagedcare.gov.au/aged-care-quality-standards
- www.health.gov.au/resources/publications/aged-care-diversity-framework
- www.myagedcare.gov.au/sites/default/files/2020-01/charter-of-aged-care-rights-booklet-english.pdf
- www.agedcareguide.com.au/information/consumer-directed-care

Role of social work:

- www.aasw.asn.au/practitioner-resources/practice-standards
- www.aasw.asn.au/practitioner-resources/code-of-ethics

Issues to consider:

- www.publicadvocate.vic.gov.au
- www.vcat.vic.gov.au
- www2.health.vic.gov.au/hospitals-and-health-services/patient-care/end-of-life-care/advance-care-planning/acp-forms

Family violence:

- www.vic.gov.au/maram-practice-guides-and-resources
- www.vic.gov.au/family-violence-information-sharing-scheme
- www.thewomens.org.au/health-professionals/clinical-resources/strengthening-hospitals-response-to-family-violence
- www.nari.net.au/primary-prevention-of-family-violence

Mental health:

- https://seniorsrights.org.au/your-rights
- www.beyondblue.org.au/who-does-it-affect/older-people/signs-and-symptoms-of-depression-in-older-people

Assessment:

- www2.health.vic.gov.au/ageing-and-aged-care/residential-aged-care/safety-and-quality/improving-resident-care/comprehensive-health-assessment
- www.nari.net.au/improving-aged-care-assessments

References

Australian Association of Social Workers. (2020). *Scope of Social Work Practice – Hospitals*. Melbourne: Australian Association of Social Workers. Retrieved from www.aasw.asn.au/document/item/8644.

Australian Government. (2016). Aged Care. Retrieved from www.aihw.gov.au/aged-care.

Australian Institute of Health and Welfare. (2014). *Australia's Health 2014*. Canberra: Australian Institute of Health and Welfare. Retrieved from www.aihw.gov.au/getmedia/19dbc591-b1ef-4485-80ce-029ff66d6930/6_9-health-ageing.pdf.aspx.

Australian Institute of Health and Welfare. (2018). Older Australia at a Glance. Retrieved from www.aihw.gov.au/reports/older-people/older-australia-at-a-glance/contents/demographics-of-older-australians/australia-s-changing-age-and-gender-profile.

Australian Institute of Health and Welfare. (2021). *Aged Care*. Canberra: Australian Institute of Health and Welfare.

Beyond Blue. (2009). *Depression in Older Age: A Scoping Study*. Final Report. Melbourne: National Aging Research Institute.

Cleak, H. & Turczynski, M. (2014). Hospital Social Work in Australia: Emerging Trends. *Social Work in Health Care*, 53(3), 199–213.

Duckett, S., Cuddihy, M. & Newnham, H. (2016). *Targeting Zero: Supporting the Victorian Hospital System to Eliminate Avoidable Harm and Strengthen Quality of Care*. Melbourne: Victorian Government. Retrieved from www2.health.vic.gov.au/hospitals-and-health-services/quality-safety-service/hospital-safety-and-quality-review.

Eastern Health. (2021). Geriatric Evaluation and Management at Home. Retrieved from www.easternhealth.org.au/services/item/555-geriatric-evaluation-and-management-at-home.

Fisk, M., Livingstone, A. & Pit, S. (2020). Telehealth in the Context of COVID-19: Changing Perspectives in Australia, the United Kingdom, and the United States. *Journal of Medical Internet Research*, 22(6), 2–13.

Fiske, A., Loebach Wetherall, J. & Gatz, M. (2009). Depression in Older Adults. *Annual Review of Clinical Psychology*, 5(1), 363–389.

Macri, J. (2016). Australia's Health System: Some Issues and Challenges. *Journal Health and Medical Economics*, 2(2).

McCallum, J. & Rees, K. (2017). *Consumer Directed Care in Australia: Early Stage Analysis and Future Directions*. Brisbane: National Seniors Australia. Retrieved from https://agedcare.royalcommission.gov.au/system/files/2020-06/NSA.9999.0006.0001.pdf.

Nicol, E. D., Mohanna, K. & Cowpe, J. (2014). Perspectives on Clinical Leadership: A Qualitative Study Exploring the Views of Senior Healthcare Leaders in the UK. *Journal of the Royal Society of Medicine*, 107(7), 277–286.

Nilsson, D. & Braddy, L. (2009). Health. In H. Cleak (ed.), *Assessment and Report Writing in the Human Services* (pp. 99–115). Victoria: Cengage Learning Australia.

Northern Health. (2021). Geriatric Evaluation and Management Program (GEM@Home). Retrieved from www.nh.org.au/service/geriatric-evaluation-management-program-gem-home/.

Office of the Public Advocate, Victoria. (2020). *Guardianship Guide – A Guide for Guardians Appointed under the Guardianship and Administration Act 2019*. Melbourne: Office of the Public Advocate, State of Victoria. Retrieved from www.publicadvocate.vic.gov.au/joomlatools-files/docman-files/booklet/Guardianship_Guide.pdf.

Parliamentary Library. (2021). Health. Retrieved from www.aph.gov.au/About_Parliament/Parliamentary_Departments/Parliamentary_Library/pubs/rp/BudgetReview201920/Health.

Sansoni, J. E., Samsa, P. D., Owen, A. G., Eagar, K. & Grootemaat, P. E. (2012). *An Assessment Framework for Aged Care*. Woolongong: Centre for Health Service Development, University of Wollongong. Retrieved from https://documents.uow.edu.au/content/groups/public/@web/@chsd/documents/doc/uow194617.pdf

Travis, D. (2015). *Travis Review Increasing the Capacity of the Victorian Public Hospital System for Better Patient Outcomes*. Melbourne: Victorian Government.

Victorian Government. (2016). More Support for Hospitals to Tackle Family Violence. Retrieved from www.premier.vic.gov.au/more-support-for-hospitals-to-tackle-family-violence/.

Victorian Government Health Hub. (2016). Screening and Assessment. Retrieved from www2.health.vic.gov.au/hospitals-and-health-services/patient-care/older-people/comm-topics/assessment.

World Health Organization. (2016). Ageing and Life-Course. Retrieved from www.who.int/ageing/publications/active/en/.

World Health Organization. (2021). Ageing and Health. Retrieved from www.who.int/news-room/fact-sheets/detail/ageing-and-health.

9 Engaging with Mental Health and Substance Use Recovery

Dual Diagnosis Practice Principles and Tools

Simon Kroes and Kevan Myers

The co-occurrence of substance use and mental health across the Australian population is very common. You will know people with these issues in your personal and professional life. In order to be effective, workers need to develop knowledge, confidence and skills in this area so that service user and carer needs are appropriately addressed. The basic principles of a dual diagnosis approach can be grasped early in practice and aligns with social work practice principles. When working with people with substance use and mental health issues, we need to be aware that stigma compounds both areas. This chapter outlines a dual diagnosis approach and provides examples based on practice wisdom from the field over many decades.

What Is 'Dual Diagnosis'?

Both nationally and internationally, a variety of terms, including 'comorbid mental health and substance use' and 'co-occurring mental health and substance use', have been used to describe the common scenario of a person having both a mental health and substance use problem (Roberts, 2013; Staiger et al., 2008; Allsop, 2008; Schulte et al., 2010; Minkoff & Cline, 2004). While recognising each of these terms bring a range of possible interpretations, this chapter will predominately use the term 'dual diagnosis' to describe the co-occurrence of mental health and substance use problems, as at the time of writing this is the commonly used term by government-funded initiatives such as the Victorian Dual Diagnosis Initiative where the authors are currently employed.

In addition to service users who have severe mental health and substance use issues, a range of dual diagnosis presentations exist. For example some people may find that:

- Caffeine increases anxiety.
- Alcohol reduces auditory hallucinations.
- Opiates numb trauma.

Given these all too common interactions, all service users should be individually screened, assessed and provided with treatment choices around the interaction between their mental health and substance use to collaboratively determine the best way to improve their quality of life.

Prevalence: Why Dual Diagnosis is the Expectation not the Exception

Internationally and within Australia, the recognition of the significance of dual diagnosis has grown over the past 20 years. For example:

DOI: 10.4324/9781003330745-11

> There is a high prevalence of substance use disorders (SUDs; including alcohol and drug abuse and dependence) among people with psychotic disorders and other serious mental illnesses, including schizophrenia, schizoaffective disorder, bipolar disorder, and major depression. Although the lifetime prevalence of SUDs in the general population is approximately 15%, about 50% of people with a psychotic disorder develop a drug or alcohol use disorder at some point in their lives.
>
> (Mueser & Gingerich, 2013, pp. 424–439)

The early mortality in people with severe mental illness (25 years earlier than individuals in the general population) is largely attributable to medical illnesses that are associated with substance use such as alcohol and tobacco. Stigma from health care professionals negatively impacts on treatments offered (Van Boekel et al., 2015). Health workers can improve outcomes by being aware of their own biases and use recovery language. Service users shouldn't be denied treatment that would be normally offered.

Australia's Response

In the late 1990s, the National Drug Strategy and National Mental Health Strategy developed the 'National Comorbidity Project' (Teesson & Burns, 2001). These initiatives were informed by international literature regarding the extent of co-morbidity experienced by people suffering from mental illness and using alcohol and other drugs, and the problems with parallel treatment systems (Drake, Mercer-McFadden, Mueser, McHugo & Bond, 1998), and have continued to note findings from overseas (SAMHSA, 2002). The Victorian Dual Diagnosis Initiative (VDDI), of which Nexus Dual Diagnosis Consultation Service is a component part, commenced in 2000. Similar initiatives were developed in other states in Australia (NSW Health 2000; Pennebaker, Robinson, Gomes, Quigley, Bennetts & Browton, 2001).

It's easy to assume that dual diagnosis only refers to consumers who have severe mental health and substance use issues. In practice, however, a range of dual diagnosis presentations exist.

Victorian Dual Diagnosis Response

In many services funded by the Victorian Department of Health dual diagnosis policy is stated as core business. The purpose of the Victorian Dual Diagnosis Initiative (Allsop, 2008) is to promote development of a systematic and integrated approach to service provision, so people of any age experiencing dual diagnosis have prompt access to quality treatment and support, focused on recovery. VDDI services provide a balance of direct care, consultation and support to primary care and other sectors working with people experiencing dual diagnosis (which would include housing, employment, education, and community organisations). Service users and families/ carers were to be involved in policy and service development both centrally and locally to enable services to be easier to use, seen as useful and aligned with their needs. Many of these elements were captured in a seminal document by the Victorian State Government in 2007 called 'Key directions and priorities for service development'. More recent documents such as the Productivity Commission Inquiry into Mental Health (Productivity Commission, 2020) and the Royal Commission into Victoria's mental health system (State of Victoria, 2021) further confirm the need for dual diagnosis issues to be adequately addressed.

A Multi-layered Response

Achieving good dual diagnosis practice relies on seven key elements. In this section, we look at each of these framework 'cornerstones', concluding with ~~the~~ parallels between these approaches and the AASW Practice Standards.

Core Business

A young man who is seeking assistance from a housing agency who has a history of homelessness stemming for childhood abuse is highly at risk of developing mental health and substance use issues. While the primary presenting need is around housing, unmet need around substance use and mental health are likely to impact on the sustainability of any housing options. Thus this provides an opportunity to explore and where possible offer interventions or referral advice.

The prevalence of dual diagnosis means social workers should approach all service users as if dual diagnosis is core business no matter where you are working. While you are likely to have a range of different capacities in terms of interventions and roles depending on your position you should consider dual diagnosis as being 'the expectation not the exception' (Minkoff & Cline, 2004). In practical terms this means when working with service users, you should be looking for emerging or existing mental health and substance use issues and have at least a basic understanding of how to screen and assess for these issues and interventions that may offered. Good professional practice calls for 'assertive treatment of comorbid substance use … (as) part of every treatment plan' (Galletly et al., 2016).

'No Wrong Door'

The myriad and complex service systems that service users with a dual diagnosis could look to for assistance are difficult to navigate. This is also often the case for health and welfare workers. One of the major difficulties for service users and their carers (family members or other support people) is the struggle to find appropriate and accepting services. The experience of being rejected from service provision has been very common with this often being couched in terms of 'we can't help you with your mental health until you until you deal with your substance use'. At worst this can mean individuals don't receive treatment for long periods which in turn worsens their prognosis as they lose other social supports. For example, we know the longer psychosis is untreated the harder it is to successfully treat. For the individual and their families, reducing the gap between first symptoms and treatment, early intervention, is vitally important. This is magnified in dual diagnosis where service users may experience being pushed from one service sector to another. The term 'no wrong door', has been popularised to improve service responsiveness. This recognises service users can and will appear in numerous service sectors and that services have a responsibility to support and guide service users to find services appropriate for their needs (Clark et al., 2008).

Person and Family Centred

Dual diagnosis practice should be person and family-centred however the history of service system response often does not articulate how this actually happens in day-to-day practice.

Service user-professional relationships should aim at a therapeutic alliance, which combines the living and lived experience knowledge of the service user and their carer with professional knowledge with an understanding of power dynamics that potentially exist. In most cases, and to the greatest degree possible, the aim should be to have the service user involved in their own treatment planning. Service users cannot develop and direct all treatment decisions in a vacuum. Workers have at their disposal a range of skills and information that would not necessarily be available to service users. Health professionals also hold a duty of care to individuals, family and the wider community, which may play a role in individual service user decision making. An example of a resource which may assist with this process is 'Carers Can Ask' (see below).

Integrated Treatment

Integrated treatment is where the service user has one plan, which includes all their concerns; mental health, substance use, housing, legal and physical health issues to ensure continuity of care with effective communication between service providers, service users and carers.

Integrated treatment is different from the concept of integrated services where numerous service types exist within one organisation. While this can deliver integrated treatment, it is not the only model for doing so.

Integrated treatment recognises that the service user remains an integrated person even when they have multiple treatment providers. Furthermore, that mental health, substance use and physical health are mutually tri-directional influencers and therefore need to be addressed in an integrated plan.

What does integrated treatment mean in practice?

- Recognition that mental health and substance use influence each other – they are bi-directional at all times.
- Mental health and substance use are both viewed as 'primary issues'.
- Treatment planning takes into account the needs of the person in relation to both issues simultaneously as opposed to parallel or sequential treatment.
- Consumers may require a number of specialist services, however where there is more than one service provider, regular communication using either one shared treatment plan or sharing of treatment plans maximises continuity of care.

Welcoming, Responsiveness and Hope

Minkoff & Cline (2004), describe a key starting point for dual diagnosis capability is how welcoming a service is when first approached by service users and their carers. Mental illness and substance use are both areas with a strong history of judgemental thinking and stigma. Service users who often experience rejection are reluctant to open up for fear of further rejection by services. In the case of service users who use illicit drugs there may be legal ramifications to consider also. Service users and carers sometimes learn by bitter experience the need to carefully tell their story in order to fit with service practice or in some cases prescribed eligibility criteria. There are a number of legal and policy documents such as the Victorian Mental Health act 2014 and the Royal Commission into

Victoria's Mental Health System (State of Victoria, 2021) which support a welcoming assertive approach.

How service users are welcomed into conversations around dual diagnosis therefore becomes a critical issue. Our experience however is that this is not as hard as it may appear. The first step is to recognise the main fear of service users is that you might be judgemental and stigmatising in your response. Secondly, the fear is that you might ignore their views and try to force them into following your prescriptions for change. Probably the best guide to welcoming is to consider how you like to be treated. Although we all have different expectations stemming from our own cultural bases there are some common factors such as being shown respect, characterised by being listened to, having our needs considered when making plans, not assuming that there is a shared understanding of an issue and being courteous.

Key resources to provide to service users and their carers are 'Consumers Can Ask' (a resource developed by Kroes in 2016) and 'Carers Can Ask' (a resource developed by Kroes in 2012). Providing these resources emphasises they not only have permission, and are entitled, to ask questions. The resource list at the end of this chapter gives further information on these resources.

Recovery Orientated

The concept of recovery has been increasingly accepted in both mental health and AOD services (Slade, Adams & O'Hagan, 2012). Social workers should be aware that 'recovery' might not be a phrase that sits well with all service users as it has connotations with a 'disease' model (Dahl, 2014). Nevertheless, the concept of recovery has been generally empowering for service users and carers. Although there are a number of definitions of recovery, they generally overlap in particular areas. Some examples include the following:

The National Framework for Recovery-Oriented Mental Health Services defines personal recovery as being able to create and live a meaningful and contributing life in a community of choice with or without the presence of mental health issues (Australian Health Ministers' Advisory Council, 2013). Recovery-oriented approaches sit within the harm minimisation framework, acknowledging and building on people's own resilience and resources. Recovery-oriented approaches recognise that people come to treatment through many different paths and that their goals and journey towards recovery and wellbeing are individual and unique.

Harm Minimisation

Harm minimisation policy has informed Australia's drug treatment strategy since 1985 (Commonwealth of Australia, Department of Health, 2017). Its goal is to lessen the negative health, societal, and economic effects of alcohol and/or other drug use without completely eradicating use (Wodak & Saunders, 1995).

There are three elements to harm minimisation:

- Supply reduction – i.e. restricting sales, border control.
- Demand reduction – i.e. general population advertising, drink/drug driving laws.
- Harm reduction – e.g. needle and syringe programmes, having water available at dance venues.

Harm reduction is a great way to engage with service users as it sends a strong message that they are valued and empowers them to make decisions. The Before During After tool (BDA) can be used to explore harm reduction.

The Parallels with Social Work

Social work practice should be holistic and multi-layered. This requires of the social worker a sense of working towards better outcomes for service users from numerous angles. This can encompass individual service user and family work, system level engagement and advocating around cultural and stigma issues. The dual diagnosis approach described in this chapter mirrors the approach of the Australian Association of Social Workers (2013) in their| practice standards.

Internationally, the International Federation of Social Workers (2014) note in their 'global definition of social work':

> principles of social justice, human rights, collective responsibility and respect for diversities are central to social work. Underpinned by theories of social work, social sciences, humanities and indigenous knowledge, social work engages people and structures to address life challenges and enhance wellbeing.

The authors have and continue to be involved in dual diagnosis capability on multiple levels.

Examples of Systems Approach in Practice

As part of our Nexus role we attend numerous network meetings with a variety of stakeholders. Examples of these include the NEDDY (North East Dual Diagnosis Youth), and the Yarra Drug and Health Forum (YDHF), which both meet monthly.

NEDDY was set up in 2010 and aims to develop best practice in integrated care, ultimately to improve outcomes for young people who have dual diagnosis issues. NEDDY is an established cross sector collaboration aligned with State and Federal dual diagnosis policy directives. Member agencies include clinical mental health, mental health community support services and alcohol and/or other drug services.

NEDDY brings many voices together to provide the following:

- a locally based avenue for staff to access peer support;
- improve skills and knowledge;
- foster links between programs (resulting in improved referrals);
- develop and share resources (such as the 'Carers Can Ask' resource); and
- run professional development opportunities such as cross sector case reviews and training on topics of interest.

YDHF is a community-based collaborative originally funded under the 'Drug Hot Spots' fund (Victoria Drug Policy Expert Committee, 2000). The broad membership – which includes AOD, MHCCS, and housing services among others – facilitates submissions, research and advocacy that may not be possible or appropriate for individuals or organisations. YDHF has supported the roll out of Naloxone training and distribution by Harm Reduction Victoria and partnered research on public injecting with the Burnet Institute (Dwyer, Power & Dietze, 2013).

Tools for Dual Diagnosis Practice

In this section, we explore various tools that can be used in everyday practice to:

- Hear a person's dual diagnosis story.
- Discuss with them interactions between their mental health and substance use.
- Identify and reflect on their reasons for substance use.
- Collaborate on treatment possibilities and encourage change.

Reasons For Use Package

The RFUP is a compilation of existing tools, interventions and information that includes the RFU scale. The RFUP also includes training material and guides for mentors and mentees. The package is built on strengths and recovery principles. It explores service user motivations in relation to their drug use and mental health and assists staff and service users to consider possible treatments or interventions.

Nexus over many years conducted meetings with various agencies, and engaged in discussions with staff, about the best ways to develop their capacity to provide evidence-based dual diagnosis treatment. Staff consistently asked for resources to assist them in developing treatment options. Staff reported they did not know, and/or did not feel confident in, how to implement or decide on the next intervention to use with service users after they have completed initial screening to detect dual diagnosis issues. In light of these discussions, Nexus was particularly interested in user-friendly interventions to assist staff in opening up dual diagnosis conversations with service users and in particular, how to link mandatory screening with interventions in a service user-centred manner.

The Reasons for Use scale (Spencer et al., 2002) had a reputation as a simple and effective engagement tool in its use as a component part of the managing mental health and substance use collaborative therapy program. To try and address the needs raised by staff, I (Simon Kroes) built a prototype dual diagnosis resource based on what I perceived to be a user friendly questionnaire or scale that was already in use that service users engaged with. Relevant skills of the field were also considered because I wanted to build a tool that could be relatively easy to train staff in and implement. A key research and practice question was 'What type of tool would assist staff to quickly start to address dual diagnosis issues?'

I put the prototype out for consultation to his team. Colleague Kevan Myers came on board and we further developed the tool and added a mentoring process to further facilitate implementation as we have found that training alone does not usually produce practice change. From inception the tool was based firmly on practice wisdom. We then sought to see if this tool did what we thought it would do and lead to the research we conducted in partnership with Neami National and Monash University in 2015. Through this process staff told us that the Reasons for Use Package was easy to use, effective in building staff and service user confidence in working with dual diagnosis issues and is one of the simplest ways to build dual diagnosis into core practice.

How you use the package is as important, if not more important, than the contents of the package

The approach to using the package is a fundamental aspect of it. How you use the package is as important, if not more important, than the contents of the package. We continually encourage staff to be curious, supportive and to explore issues with the service user in a non-judgemental manner.

The aim of the package is to improve the quality of life of the service users which may or may not include reducing or changing their drug use. We believe that having a respectful conversation with the service user that explores their mental health and substance use and then providing and negotiating potential strategies or treatments is the best way to begin to address the sometimes complex but treatable issues that surround dual diagnosis issues.

Reflection: George's Story

George is a male in his late thirties with a 10-year history of presentations to mental health services. Diagnosis of schizophrenia, and polysubstance use including, heroin, alcohol and tobacco.

Context: George was in a Mental Health Acute Inpatient Unit

A Psychiatric Nurse facilitated the RFUP with him and he scored the following in the scale section for alcohol use:

Coping with positive symptoms and medication side effects: 9

Conformity/acceptance: 11

Coping with unpleasant affect: 24

Enhancement: 12

Social use: 7

Using the treatment planning section of the RFUP George, supported by the nurse, came up with the following treatment plan:

- Consider grounding strategies
- Medication review
- Self-help groups
- Harm reduction strategies developed using the BDA.

In the process of administering the RFUP, service user and staff member expertise is brought together, to collaboratively develop potential treatments options. The service user is at the centre of their own treatment.

The RFUP has been in use for over ten years and has been implemented nationally. It is embedded in public clinical mental health services and community support and rehabilitation services across Australia. Published articles based on the research into the RFUP are available in the reference list.

Before During After (BDA) Harm Reduction Package

The BDA tool provides a user friendly and comprehensive method for exploring harm reduction with service users. To aid implementation the full BDA package includes a variety of resources, training and mentoring, consultation, and evaluation measures. In 1995, I (Simon Kroes), developed the BDA concept and used it in practice for many years prior to working at Nexus Dual Diagnosis Consultation Service. After commencing employment with Nexus I ran an initial multi-site pilot involving 5 MHCSS sites in 2016. In 2016 a Quality

Assurance project at a Community Care Unit found the BDA increased staff knowledge and confidence about how to explore harm reduction issues with service users. Service users found the resource improves their therapeutic relationship with staff and improves their ability to develop collaborative treatment goals (Morrison, Owens, Kroes, Myers & Petrakis, 2017). It provided the organisation with a clear structure that could be measured. importantly the evidence demonstrates the ease of application and usefulness of the package.

The BDA has been implemented at a Community Care unit, a Prevention and Recovery Centre (PARC) and two mental health youth residential service.

Carers and Consumers Can Ask resources

Carers Can Ask (CCA) is a collaborative engagement tool for families, carers and clinicians designed to assist communication between carers and health services. The resource comprises questions carers can ask to find out about treatment and discharge planning and other information. Created in 2013 by Simon Kroes as a co-designed North East Dual Diagnosis Youth network (NEDDY) project utilising input from carers, consumers and staff across Victoria, the CCA has been distributed via the Caring Together and St Vincent's Hospital websites. The Independent Mental Health Advocacy Service (IMHA) and the Mental Health Complaints Commission (MHCC) have distributed it also. It has been used in practice extensively by carer consultants. Numerous hospitals across Victoria have modified it for their own geographical areas.

The CCA aligns with current strategic directions in mental health services such as the findings of the Royal Commission into Victoria's mental health system (State of Victoria, 2021) and the 4th Australian National Mental Health plan 2012 (Department of Health and Ageing, 2013).

> What a terrific resource you have created!
>
> (Carer Consultant South Australia)

Using the structure of Carers Can Ask, Kroes undertook further consultations with service users and service user consultants to develop the resource into Consumers Can Ask for service users.

> That Consumer Can Ask package would have to be the most comprehensive and relevant resource for Consumers that I have seen.
>
> (Senior peer mental health project worker)

Straight Up Lived Experience Resource

Kevan Myers was one of the project leads from Nexus who worked with Monash University Art Design & Architecture to co-produce the Straight Up.org website. The website uses animation linked to the voices of real service user and carers. It has been used effectively in training and education to assist staff and tertiary students to gain an understanding of the issues from a living/ lived experience perspective. The animations have been viewed by thousands of people since its launch in 2018.

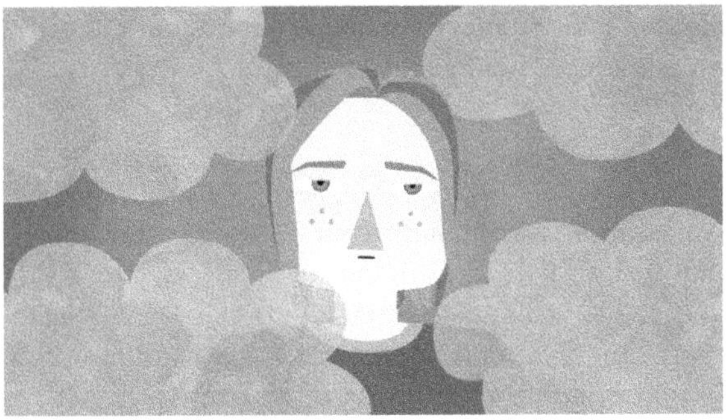

Figure 9.1 Johan
Source: Cameron Rose

Johan explains his path to addiction and recovery and how being treated like a normal human being gave him the motivation to see it through. The video of Johan can be viewed at: https://www.straightup.org.au/

Motivational Interviewing

Motivational interviewing (MI) is a form of collaborative conversation originally developed in the addictions arena and now has an evidence base for use in numerous settings including mental health, corrections and physical health.

Miller and Rollnick (2013) define MI as a person-centred, collaborative, goal-oriented style of communication which focuses particular attention on the language of change. It is designed to strengthen personal motivation and commitment to a specific goal by eliciting and exploring the person's own reasons for change within an atmosphere of acceptance and compassion. Learning MI takes time and is best achieved through a range of activities including training and reflective practice. Core elements, such as the Spirit of Motivational Interviewing, which is comprised of four elements: partnership, compassion, evocation & acceptance are within reach for those at the beginning of their practice.

Relapse Prevention

When working to change any pattern of behaviour lapse and relapse are common events. This is particularly evident when service users are trying to change substance use. Understanding and learning to manage cravings and relapse prevention are therefore key ingredients (Larimer & Marlatt, 2004).

> It is possible to understand drug craving and to learn how to manage drug craving without returning to drug use. A model that allows people to identify set-up behaviours (these are ways of thinking, managing feelings, and behaving that increase the risk of having a relapse), trigger events, and the cycle of drug craving itself, and intervening upon this process has proven effective in reducing relapse.
>
> (Gorski, 2001)

Wellness Recovery Action Plans (WRAP) have also been found to be of assistance in reducing the likelihood of relapse for service users with a dual diagnosis (St Vincent's,

2014). The main aim of this type of document is to build understanding of possible relapse triggers and plan supports to mitigate them.

Conclusion

Social workers are very likely to come into contact with people who have or are likely to develop a dual diagnosis. It is incumbent on all social workers that they should work towards having a basic dual diagnosis capacity so that rather than being a barrier to recovery they can support individuals, carers and the community as a whole to create an environment within which hope is maintained and recovery becomes the expectation. There are a range of evidence based tools and resources that can be useful when working with a person who has a dual diagnosis. Social workers should look for opportunities to work for system change through advocacy and networking to reduce the negative impacts of stigma and create environments which facilitate better outcomes for service users with a dual diagnosis and their cares.

- Dual diagnosis is common but treatable.
- Dual diagnosis is any impact drug use has on mental health, and any impact mental health has on drug use.
- The natural progression is for a person to trend toward recovery.
- Understanding and talking through reasons for use can be empowering for the service user and create meaningful treatment pathways.
- There are evidence-based interventions for dual diagnosis that can aid individuals and carers on their recovery journeys.

Reflection Questions

How will you be welcoming and non-judgemental when working with service users with a dual diagnosis and their carers?

What tools and approaches do you think you will use in practice?

How will you make a dual diagnosis approach part of your core practice?

Key Website Resources

Nexus, St Vincent's Hospital Fitzroy Victoria, Australia (https://svhm.org.au/home/our-services/departments-and-services/n/nexus).

Straight Up (www.straightup.org.au and www.svhm.org.au/our-services/departments-and-services/n/nexus/straight-up).

BDA link (www.svhm.org.au/our-services/departments-and-services/n/nexus/bda).

RFUP link (www.svhm.org.au/our-services/departments-and-services/n/nexus/resources/rfu-package and https://reasonsforusepackage.com).

CCA link (www.svhm.org.au/our-services/departments-and-services/n/nexus/carers-can-ask).

References

Allsop, S. (2008) *Drug Use and Mental Health.* IP Communications Melbourne.

Australian Association of Social Workers. (2013). *Practice Standards.* Canberra: AASW.

Australian Health Ministers' Advisory Council. (2013). *A National Framework for Recovery-Oriented Mental Health Services: Guide for Practitioners and Providers*. Australian Health Ministers' Advisory Council.

Best, D. W. & Lubman, D. I. (2012). The recovery paradigm: A model of hope and change for alcohol and drug addiction. *Australian Family Physician*, 41(8), 593.

Byrne,L., Happell, B. & Reid-Searl, K. (2015). *Lived Experience Practitioners and the Medical Model: Worlds Colliding*. Journal of Mental Health.

Clark, H. W., Power, A. K., Le Fauve, C.E. & Lopez, E. I. (2008). Policy and practice implications of epidemiological surveys on co-occurring mental and substance use disorders. *Journal of Substance Abuse Treatment*, 34(1), 3–13.

Commonwealth of Australia, Department of Health. (2017). *National Drug Strategy 2017–2026*. Commonwealth of Australia, Department of Health.

Corrigan, P. (2004). How stigma interferes with mental health care. *American Psychologist*, 59(7), 614.

Dahl, S. L. (2014). Remaining a user while cutting down: The relationship between cannabis use and identity. Retrieved from http://informahealthcare.com/doi/abs/10.3109/09687637.2014.920765

Department of Health (2012). *Psychiatric Disability and Rehabilitation and Support Services Reform Framework Consultation Paper – Consultation Report*. Melbourne: State Government of Victoria.

Department of Health and Ageing (2013) *National Mental Health Report 2013: tracking progress of mental health reform in Australia 1993 – 2011*. Canberra: Commonwealth of Australia.

Department of Human Services (2007). *Dual Diagnosis – Key Directions and Priorities for Service Development*. Melbourne: State Government of Victoria.

Drake, R. E., Mercer-McFadden, C., Mueser, K. T., McHugo, G. J. & Bond, G. R. (1998). Review of integrated mental health and substance treatment for patients with dual disorders. *Schizophrenia Bulletin*, 24(4), 589–608.

Dwyer, R., Power, R. & Dietze, P. (2013). North Richmond Public Injecting Impact Study Community report. Retrieved from www.burnet.edu.au/system/asset/file/1043/Report-Nth_Richmond_Public_Injecting_Impact.pdf.

Galletly, C., Castle, D., Dark, F., Humberstone, V., Jablensky, A., Killackey, E., Kulkarni, J., McGorry, P., Nielssen, O. & Tran, N. (2016). Royal Australian and New Zealand College of Psychiatrists clinical practice guidelines for the management of schizophrenia and related disorders. *Australian & New Zealand Journal of Psychiatry*, 50(5), pp.410–472.

Gorski. T. T. (2001). Cocaine, craving, and relapse. Retrieved from www.tgorski.com/orski_articles/cocaine%20craving%20&%20relapse%20010523.htm.

Hartz, S. M., Pato, C. N., Medeiros, H., Cavazos-Rehg, P., Sobell, J. L., Knowles, J. A., ... & Vivar, A. (2014). Comorbidity of severe psychotic disorders with measures of substance use. *JAMA Psychiatry*, 2014.

International Federation of Social Workers. (2014). *Global definition of social work*. In IFSW General Meeting and the IASSW General Assembly.

Kavanagh, D. (2020). *Productivity Commission Inquiry into Mental Health*. Queensland University of Technology.

Kroes, S., Myers, K., Officer, S., O'Connor, S. & Petrakis, M. (2019). Dual diagnosis assessment: A case study implementing the reasons for use package to engage a marginalised service user. *Cogent Medicine*, 6(1), 1630097.

Larimer, M. E. & Marlatt, G. A. (2004). Relapse prevention: An overview of Marlatt's cognitive-behavioral model. *Psychosocial Treatments*, 2004, 11–28.

Miller, W. R. & Rollnick, S. (2013) *Motivational Interviewing; Helping People Change*. Guildford Press.

Mills, K., Marel, C., Madden, E. & Teeson, M. (2019). Lessening the burden of comorbid substance use and mental disorders through evidence-based care: The case for a national minimum qualifications strategy. Retrieved from www.pc.gov.au/__data/assets/pdf_file/0003/240798/ sub280-mental-health.pdf.

Minkoff, K & Cline, C (2004). Changing the world: The design and implementation of comprehensive continuous integrated systems of care for individuals with co-occurring disorders. *Psychiatric Clinics of North America*, 27, 4.

Morrison, B., Owens, C., Kroes, S. E., Myers, K. & Petrakis, M. (2017). *Before during after: A harm reduction tool.* Mental Health Services (MHS) Conference 2017: Embracing Change: Through Innovation and Lived Experience. August.

Mueser, K. T. & Gingerich, S. (2013). Treatment of co-occurring psychotic and substance use disorders. *Social Work in Public Health*, 28, 424–439.

Myers, K., Kroes, S., O'Connor, S. & Petrakis, M. (2020). Reasons for use package: Outcomes from a case comparison evaluation. *Research on Social Work Practice*, 30(7), 783–790.

NSW Health. (2000). *The Management of People with a Co-existing Mental Health and Substance Use Disorder – Service Delivery Guidelines.* Sydney: NSW Health Department.

Pennebaker, D., Robinson, S., Gomes, A., Quigley, A., Bennetts, A. & Browton, R. (2001). *Co-occurring Mental Illness and Substance Abuse Services Review.* West Perth, Western Australia: Centre for Mental Health Services Research.

Petrakis, M., Robinson, R., Myers, K., Kroes, S. & O'Connor, S. (2018). Dual diagnosis competencies: A systematic review of staff training literature. *Addictive Behaviors Reports*, 7, 53–57.

Prochaska, J. O. & DiClemente, C. C. (1984). *The Transtheoretical Approach: Crossing Traditional Boundaries of Therapy.* Homewood, IL: Dow/Jones Irwin.

Productivity Commission. (2020). *Mental Health.* Report no. 95. Canberra: Australian Federal Government.

Reason, P. & Bradbury, H. (eds). (2001). *Handbook of Action Research: Participative Inquiry and Practice.* London: Sage Publications.

Roberts, B. (2013). The seeds of dual diagnosis discourse in an Australian state. *Mental Health and Substance Use*, 6(4).

Rose, C., Myers, K., Kroes, S., Gugliemetti, M. & Hwang, I. D. (2018). *Reasons For Use Package Online.* St Vincent's Hospital Fitzroy Victoria, Australia.

SAMHSA. (2002). *Report to Congress on the Prevention and Treatment of Co-occurring Substance Abuse and Mental Disorders.* Rockville, MD: Substance Abuse and Mental Health Services Administration (SAMHSA).

Schulte, S., Meier, P., Stirling, J. & Berry, M. (2010). Dual diagnosis competency among addiction treatment staff: Training levels, training needs and the link to retention. *European Addiction Research*, 16, 78–84.

Slade, M., Adams, N. & O'Hagan, M. (2012). Recovery: past progress and future challenges. *International Review of Psychiatry*, 24(1), 1–4.

Spencer, C., Castle, D. & Michie, P.T. (2002). Motivations that maintain substance use among individuals with psychotic disorders. *Schizophrenia Bulletin*, 28(2), 233–247.

Staiger, P. *et al.* (2008) *Consumers with a Dual Diagnosis: To What Extent Do They Fall Through the Net.* Deakin University & Southern Health.

State of Victoria. (2021). *Royal Commission into Victoria's Mental Health System.* State of Victoria.

St Vincent's. (2014). *The Strengths Model: A Recovery-Oriented Approach to Mental Health Services.* Melbourne: St Vincent's Hospital.

Teesson, M. & Burns, L. (eds). (2001). *National Drug Strategy and National Mental Health Strategy, National Comorbidity Project.* Canberra: Commonwealth Department of Health and Aged Care.

Teeson, M. & Proudfoot, H. (2003). *Comorbid Mental Disorders and Substance Use Disorders: Epidemiology, Prevention and Treatment.* National Drug and Alcohol Research Centre (NDARC), University of New South Wales, Australia.

Van Boekel, L. C., Brouwers, E. P., van Weeghel, J. & Garretsen, H. F. (2015). Stigma among health professionals towards patients with substance use disorders and its consequences for healthcare delivery: systematic review. *Tijdschrift voor psychiatrie*, 57(7).

Victoria Drug Policy Expert Committee. (2000). *Drugs: Responding to the Issues, Engaging the Community. Stage One Report*. Design + Production: AD [ART] DESIGN.

Wodak, A. & Saunders W. (1995). Harm reduction means what I choose it to mean. *Drug Alcohol Review*, 14, 269–271.

10 Social Work Practice and People Living with Disability

Niki Edwards and Julie King

Introduction

Disability is a deeply personal experience that means different things to different people. How disability is defined is evolving and changing. Typically understood through a biomedical lens with regard to the impact of impairments on a person's independent life in the community; disability is broadly considered a global and universal phenomenon. This chapter examines disability at international, national and personal levels. The power of language is considered given a medicalised Global North problem-saturated grand narrative of disability has emerged. This approach is entrenched in contemporary social work practice; hence the need for critical examination and reflexivity. Potential contributions of the critical social worker will be outlined and expanded upon.

The Global Context

Disability is socially constructed, imbued with meaning in different ways by different cultures, and very far from a heterogenous experience (Grech & Soldatic, 2016; Munyi, 2012). The varied experiences of living with impairments that some describe as disability should be simply considered part of the diversity of being human (Deleuze, 1997; Overboe, 2012). However, there is a tendency to focus on binaries about what is 'normal' and what is 'abnormal' (Leshota & Sefotho, 2020); and linked categorisations of intelligence, body functionality, health status or how the 'ordinary' person thinks or acts along of a continuum of sub-average through to above average (Davis, 2010).

The first and currently only world report on disability produced by the World Health Organization (WHO) and the World Bank highlights that more than one billion people across the world live with physical, sensory, psychosocial or cognitive impairments (WHO & World Bank, 2011). This report relied on a blend of quality and projected data; hence it is likely to underestimate the prevalence of disability. Regardless, the magnitude of disability and the impact on individuals, families, communities and more broadly society is growing. It is erroneous to think living with disability is a minority issue. Globally 15% of the population are estimated to have a disability and the majority (i.e., approximately 80% live in Global South, notably in developing countries) (WHO & World Bank, 2011). It is important to recognise that the driving forces behind theory and understanding of disability have focused on the experiences of people from the Global North (i.e. Western world views) (Katsui & Swartz, 2021; Swartz, 2019; Grech & Soldatic, 2016). Caution must be exercised given

DOI: 10.4324/9781003330745-12

there is no evidence of the universality of understanding of disability using Global North perspectives. In fact, impairment should be deconstructed in context of neoliberalism, colonialism, capitalism and patriarchy that have influenced Global South approaches to disability (Connell, 2011).

Critical social workers must be alert to assumptions that Global North experiences of disability somehow 'erase' the experiences of local people with disability or more particularly, Indigenous peoples (Velarde, 2018). Government and policy makers around the world have been encouraged by the WHO and World Bank to 'step up' to disability; urging efforts to enable access to mainstream services and invest in specialised programmes to unlock the potential of people with disability (WHO & World Bank, 2011). This is consistent with the United Nations Convention on the Rights of Persons with Disabilities (UNCRPD) that focuses on the protection of human rights and empowerment of people with disability to access and enjoy full citizenship.

In Australia, approximately 1 in 6 or 18% of the population (about 4.4 million) report living with disability (Australian Institute of Health and Welfare, 2020). The Australian Bureau of Statistics (Australian Bureau of Statistics, 2019) advise that a further 22% of Australians live with a long-term health condition but no disability, and the remaining 60% have no disability or long-term health condition. For about 3 in 4 (77%) people with disability, their main form of disability (their main condition or the one causing the most problems) is physical; and for the remaining 1 in 4 (23%), their main form of disability is mental, intellectual/developmental or behavioural including mental illness (Australian Bureau of Statistics, 2019).

Family and carers often provide significant support for people with disability. The Australian Bureau of Statistics reported in 2018 that 10.8% of all Australians were carers; most carers are female, and seven in ten (71.8%) primary carers were women (Temple et al., 2018). Disability impacts not only people with impairments but also their families, friends, communities and society. Neoliberal governments conceptualise disability as an individual issue (i.e. a personal or private obligation and responsibility). Nonetheless, if disability is an 'ordinary' part of the diversity of the human condition, there are human rights directed social obligations around full citizenship. The UNCRPD enshrines the human rights of people with disability. Key tenets underpinning this convention includes human dignity and non-discrimination, full participation, social inclusion, equality of opportunity, and accessibility (United Nations, 2006). However, people with disability can be particularly disadvantaged by healthism due to the intersection of their oppressed identities arising from social exclusion, unmet or poorly recognised healthcare needs and lower socioeconomic status (Sakellariou & Rotarou, 2017). Consistent with medicalised understanding, healthism sites the 'problem' of disability within the individual who is held responsible for 'fixing' or remedying health and social inclusion issues arising (Crawford, 1980).

People with disability face many obstacles to health and well-being, and a good quality of life. Despite protections in Australian legislation and Australia being a signatory to the UNCRPD, significant numbers of Australians with a disability continue to experience discrimination with important human capital implications (Temple et al., 2018). Stigma and discrimination are frequent features of everyday life, often fuelled by ignorance, resulting in significant distress, isolation and social exclusion (Krnjacki et al., 2017). Many people with disability and their families experience problems with access to health care, disability and community services; and a range of other serious challenges, including domestic and family violence, justice and safety issues; challenges with appropriate care arrangements including trained carers; low employment; income insecurity; insecure, unsafe or inappropriate housing, and transport barriers (Australian Institute of Health and Welfare, 2020). These issues intersect with poverty and discrimination to produce significant barriers to living a good life in contemporary society.

Human rights sit at the heart of many of these issues. Social work practice has a key role to play in this space: whether working at the micro, meso or macro levels. Critical practice obligates working for and beside people with disability to enable empowerment, social justice, equality and equity. The profession is committed to maximising the well-being of individuals, families, groups, communities and society (Australian Association of Social Workers, 2016, 2020). Social workers hold potential to make a strong contribution to this space by walking alongside and advocating for required systemic changes to enable people with disability to enjoy full citizenship: focusing on working *with* people with disability (i.e. '*nothing about us without us*' as opposed to '*doing things to*' people with disability) (Charlton, 2000).

Power of Language

Communication and use of language is shaped by history, philosophy and politics (O'Brien, 2010). A common childhood chant was 'sticks and stones will break my bones but names will never hurt me'. How untrue! Language is powerful. When people think about or discuss disability they may resort to historical terms that are imbued with negativity. An ableist belief system often underpins such negative attitudes, stereotypes and stigma toward people with disability. Ableism includes ideas, practices, institutions, and social relations that presume perfect abled bodies; therefore, constructing and othering people with disability who may be marginalised and mostly invisible (Chouinard et al., 2016). Ableism captures negative attitudes in society that devalue and limit the potential of persons with disability.

Highly stigmatised words that reflect privileging of ableism and describe people with disability still abound in school playgrounds, workplaces, recreational activities and media stories (Linton, 2010; Pelleboer-Gunnink et al., 2021). It is not uncommon but highly inappropriate and discriminatory to hear the terms 'retard', 'idiot' or 'spastic'. These pejorative and harmful descriptors can be historically linked to outdated diagnostic labels used for people with intellectual disability and physical disability. For example, impairment associated with mental illness, more recently reconceptualised as psychosocial disability, has influenced many words, including 'insane', 'mad', and 'loony'. These words are far from innocuous, use can be conceptualised as microaggressions and they powerfully perpetrate negative and inappropriate stereotypes and unjustly reduce disability to a negative experience (Olkin et al., 2019).

Social workers need to take care with language and descriptions and recognise that the neoliberal grand narrative of disability is resilient and persistent; it has been influenced by biomedical models and simplistically reduced disability to a 'problem' in need of restoration and preferably cure. However, disability is an intensely personal and individualised experience. Critical social workers must respect the uniqueness, voice and agency of individuals living with disability. While it is important to be familiar with key definitions of disability and impairment, it should be noted that there is no consensus and definitions remain contested and disputed (Chenoweth, 2017).

Critical Self-Reflection about Disability

This is an exercise that you should not spend too much time thinking about – simply do it, practice deconstruction and reconstruction. Then reflect and think deeply about what came to mind; what you thought about; what comes to mind when you respond to the question.

Task

> Close your eyes and think 'disability'. What mental image comes to mind? Take a snapshot of that image. Describe that image in some detail – taking care not to describe what you think disability should look like but describe that image that quickly came to mind.

Response

Most people tend to 'see' or conceptualise a person with a physical disability: typically, a person in a wheelchair. This is not surprising given the accessibility image of a person in wheelchair that is the symbol for disability in the Global North and now the Global South. People with physical disability have been strong advocates for change over time. However, disability is very diverse and far from homogenous. Typically, Global North conceptualisations of disability identify that there are four types of impairment experienced by people living with disability: physical impairment sensory impairment (hearing and sight impairment); psychosocial impairment (mental illness); and cognitive impairment (intellectual/ developmental disability and cognitive disability secondary to brain injury). It is imperative that critical social workers recognise this conceptualisation reinforces the dominance of the Global North grand narrative of disability that is problem saturated and linked to the medical model. Despite focus on the social model of disability and human rights-based approaches to disability in legislation, policy and ideology of many different services inclusive of health care; people with disability should be empowered to articulate their own understanding of their 'disability' or 'impairments', such as how they embody and embrace their diversity, and how they wish to live their lives.

Contemporary Definitions of Disability

Disability then can be understood as a complex, dynamic, multidimensional, and contested issue and experience (WHO & World Bank, 2011, p. 3). Really a label and often a diagnosis; disability involves deeply personal experiences arising from the intersection between health conditions, personal factors, social-cultural and environmental factors. Social workers must seek the personal narrative as a resource for responsive and informed practice (Bishop & Sunderland, 2013; Thill, 2019). It is important to analyse definitions that can influence service access and uptake. Definitions can be used to gate keep service access or allocate resources and funds. Traditionally, 'traditional' categories of disability include physical impairment; sensory Impairment; intellectual/cognitive Impairment; and psychosocial impairment. The preamble of the UNCRPD articulates a useful contemporary definition: it recognises that disability is an evolving concept; a consequence of the interaction between persons with impairments and attitudinal and environmental barriers that hinders full and effective participation in society on an equal basis with others (WHO & World Bank, 2011).

History

Understanding of disability has changed through the centuries. Leshota and Sefotho, 2020 point out that in ancient Greek, the term 'αδυνατος' meant something akin to disability and these individuals were accorded pity and charity. They discuss how the ancient Greeks and Romans focused on giving meaning to bodies; characterising what was considered normal, natural, perfect and whole. The first mental asylum can be traced back as early as the fifth century in the Middle East (Harris, 2014); prior to that families who had relatives living with disability typically provided care at home. The Industrial Revolution and urbanisation that occurred in the eighteenth and nineteenth centuries in the Global North gave families improved access to institutions and asylums that were preferred models of care at those times (Barnes, 2010). Society was 'protected' from disability and people who were considered sick or inferior were rejected, with the focus being containment as opposed to therapy, rehabilitation or empowerment (Munyi, 2012).

During the 1960s and 1970s residential and institutional care options, maintained by hospitals and health services, formed the mainstay of service provision in the Global North, including for Australians with disability (Chenoweth, 2018). However, following decades of change encouraged by disability advocates, the late twentieth century and early twenty-first century welcomed the era of community care and support (Lemay, 1995; Charlton, 2000). The leadership of people with physical disability was influential at this time, including people living with the consequences of polio and the impact of world wars (Chenoweth, 2018). For people with intellectual and developmental disability, the principals of Normalisation and Social Role Valorisation (SRV) developed by Wolfensberger strongly shaped new service approaches (Lemay, 1995); in particular, deinstutionalisation and approaches to community care (Chenoweth, 2018). These principles advocated fiercely for achievement of an enhanced level of social equality and full citizenship for people living with disability. There was significant associated debate around conceptual models of disability that shaped service development.

Conceptual Models of Disability

Medical and charity models have traditionally dominated service delivery; influenced by the grand narrative of disability. These approaches have been disputed as problem saturated and the social model of disability welcomed, later complemented by the human rights model.

Such conceptual models can seem rather abstract, but analysis is useful for many reasons:

- Identifies approaches to understanding and responding to disability.
- Informs systemic strategies responsive to needs of people with disability.
- Gives insight into societal attitudes and prejudices.
- Reveals how society, governments, communities and individuals enable or limit access to services and political power for people with disability.

There are many different 'models' of disability. However, four key models are explored due to their ongoing influence on ableist understanding and consequently Australian and international service design and delivery.

Medical Model

This model has historically shaped services including contemporary legislation, policy and program development in the Global North and the Global South. Despite significant criticism, it remains a dominant feature of contemporary health, disability and social services (Chenoweth, 2018). Disability is viewed as a problematic feature of the person, typically 'something wrong' that is caused by disease, trauma or health conditions (Oliver, 1990; Davis, 2010). This model understands that people with disability require expert medical care from doctors and allied health professionals. Healthism is evident (e.g. the person *is* the problem and is held individually responsible). Ideally cure is sought and treatment focuses on 'correcting' the problem.

Charity Model

The charity model 'sees' people with disability as 'tragic' and deserving 'victims' in need of sympathy and social care due to 'inability'. Typically people with disability are considered objects of pity. Society is positioned to feel 'sorry' for people with disability and services provide a culture of care. Charity, religious and non-government organisations have historically provided care; people with disability are expected to be grateful for the services or support (Lemay, 1995). Similar to the medical model, they are passive and dependent recipients.

Social Model

This model considers disability is created by society resulting in exclusion and disadvantage; specifically refuting disability as an attribute of the person as constructed by the medical model (Oliver, 1990). The idea of disability is re-purposed to capture external, socially created disadvantage and marginalisation experienced by people who with 'impairments' (Lawson & Beckett, 2021). Disability arises from interaction between negative social attitudes and problematic physical environments. Stigma and discrimination play powerful roles (Brown, 2010). This model mandates that as the 'problem' lies with society and the environment, society must implement relevant changes.

Human Rights Model

People with disability are increasingly active (Charlton, 2000). Their voices were heard when on 13 December 2006, the UNCRPD and the Optional Protocol were adopted by the United Nations. Two years later, 3 May 2008, it was entered into force enshrining the rights of persons with disability into a dedicated internationally persuasive human rights instrument. Australia was one of the original state signatories and on 17 July 2008 and 30 July 2009 sequentially, Australia ratified the UNCRPD and the Optional Protocol. This Convention obligates Australian governments to respect the human rights of people with disability. It signals and drives important changes in attitudes towards people with disability and their rights to social inclusion. The UNCRPD relegates the medicalised grand narrative of disability to the shadows; it shifts focus from people with disability being 'sick' and hence burdens on society or objects of charity; to recognising their rights to active full citizenship.

Disability can be conceptualised as a socio-political construct within a rights-based discourse (Degener, 2016). Profoundly influenced by the UNCRPD, this human rights model complements and improves the social model; there is sustained emphasis in shifting focus from dependence to independence (i.e. people with disability become politically active against social forces of ableism) (Lawson & Beckett, 2021). Social structures and policies restricting or ignoring the rights of people with disability often lead to discrimination and exclusion; hence, targets for change (Degener, 2016). The human rights approach requires society, particularly governments, to actively promote the necessary conditions for all individuals to fully embrace citizenship and realise their human rights.

Biopsychosocial/Spiritual/Cultural Holistic Understanding

So which model is the 'best' model and which model should critical social workers embrace? Disability is a complex phenomenon that is both an experience and challenge at the level of a person's physical being but primarily a socially constructed phenomenon. A culturally mediated category; hence, meanings of disability are shaped and influenced by the norms of the culture within which the norms exist (Leshota & Sefotho, 2020). It has already been stressed that disability is a very individual experience that involves an interaction between features of the individual and the overall context in which the person lives.

Social workers need to shift understanding of disability from a condition of 'abnormality' to embrace 'human diversity'. The French philosopher Deleuze offers useful insights here as he postulated that disability should be appreciated as a unique articulation of difference: as a dividuation of the life-force that constitutes all human beings (Deleuze, 1994). If a a Deleuzian ontology is accepted, all people are specific modifications of difference. Perhaps pause and reflect; social work welcomes, embraces and celebrates diversity and difference. A Deleuzian approach argues 'disability' per se cannot be conceived as located in a single body or subjectivity but disability is best understood as a context-specific articulation of omnipresent difference (Cockayne et al., 2017). Regardless, difference and diversity places consequent emphasis on social inclusion, equal human rights and privileges that are enjoyed by all citizens of society. The social worker's focus on person-in-environment and comprehensive ecological assessments are critical and worthy approaches when working alongside, with and in collaboration with people living with disability.

Social workers acknowledge the importance of a holistic understanding of a person within their context. In reality, dimensions of each of the models discussed above have contributions to make. A biopsychosocial/spiritual/cultural approach acknowledges that both the medical and social models need to be integrated as neither is sufficient on its own to explain the complex nature of a person's health and well-being, inclusive of disability. At the practical level, if the social worker privileges the voice and agency of the person with disability, the models provide some insights into the subjective experiences of the person who may be the client, patient or a consumer. This framework provides an essential contribution to accurate diagnosis, health outcomes, and appropriate care and requires services that enable a full and flourishing life. The attentive critical social worker who is reading this chapter will have noted the inclusion of spiritual/cultural components; to be truly holistic these domains also need careful attention. Additionally, environment should embrace both physical and social environments.

Living with Disability

Challenges for people with disability vary and this chapter has reinforced how important it is that social workers acknowledge that disability is constructed not only socially and culturally but personally (Oliver, 1990). It can also be influenced by the type of impairment that results in a disability being experienced. The voices of people with physical and sensory disability are often dominant but step back and think about how often are the voices of people with intellectual or developmental disability and individuals with psychosocial disability heard (Pilgrim & Tomasini, 2012)? Significant support may be required as a person with psychosocial disability journeys towards recovery. However, there are two active discourses that may not complement one another; limitations associated with disability versus possibilities for living well with disability (Slade & Longden, 2015; Topor et al., 2011). However, some disabilities are hidden and socially devalued; the voices of these people need to be heard and responded to given UNCRPD human rights obligations. Some of the key barriers for people with disability are:

- access, inclusion and citizenship;
- poverty;
- limited availability of services;
- policy and legislation that enables;
- physical and informational barriers;
- education;
- employment;
- attitudes and awareness;
- social and cultural beliefs; and
- stigma and discrimination.

Social and Cultural Construction of Disability

In an increasingly multicultural society and a globalised world social workers need to think carefully about the impact of society and culture on the lived experience of people with disability. When people from other cultures enter Australia they do not check their cultural beliefs in at the immigration desk. Culture is part of who people are and influences values, beliefs, ethics, morals and behaviour. While outward identifiers of culture may change, the deeply rooted values and beliefs 'held dear' are less likely to change although there is often adaption in response to new living situations (King et al. 2016).

Health and illness are influenced by social, cultural and behavioural factors and conditions, as is risk and its consequences. The same influences for disability and impairment can be assumed. Health, illness, impairment and disability therefore occur in a complex interrelationship of biological, environmental, social and cultural factors. Interpretation of social and cultural worlds shape explanations of impairment and disability and importantly, in many cultures there is no word for disability (Heneker et al., 2017; Horsell, 2020). Consequently, many people from culturally and linguistically diverse (CaLD) or where English is another language, do not identify as having a disability and lack experience in accessing support (National Ethnic and Disability Alliance, 2019). These factors are just as powerful as medical diagnoses or physical access and attitudinal barriers.

Disability may be experienced differently between cultures and this can impact on the ability of individuals and their family or carers to access services; and for services to work successfully with people from CaLD backgrounds. Findings from a 2016 study on people from refugee backgrounds living with disability in Queensland, Australia (King et al., 2016) found the following:

- Little research or known about how disability is experienced in people from refugee backgrounds.
- An unknown proportion of people from refugee backgrounds arrive with disability or disability is identified after their arrival.
- It is likely that there is an undiagnosed proportion of this population with disability as many have been subjected to torture, have lived in environments of extreme poverty, or have experienced other hardships.

Further, there is minimal research conducted around the globe that explores the lived experience of people from refugee backgrounds with disability. Similarly, the Australian experience is also relatively unknown. King and colleagues also reported that:

- Some refugees have low literacy and cannot advocate for their rights.
- Lack of language support.
- Concern for children born in Australia to parents for refugee backgrounds – cultural and language issues.
- Low familiarity with services/transport.
- Hidden or undetected disabilities (not picked up before arrival) exist.
- Lack of cultural safety.
- Inconsistent use of interpreters.
- Diversity assumed but not a homogeneous group.
- Feelings of isolation from mainstream and own communities.
- Lack of voice, agency and consequently feelings of powerlessness.
- Often interruptions to the settlement process.

(King et al., 2016)

Social Work and Disability

Social workers work with individuals, families, carers and communities. The AASW identifies key roles for practitioners including: local area coordinators, planners, community development and direct practice roles. Social workers can provide a wide range of supports including:

- therapeutic interventions and support services (individual and group);
- early intervention supports for early childhood;
- behaviour assessment and support;
- specialised assessment of skills, abilities and needs;
- assistance in coordinating or managing life stages, transitions and supports; and
- assistance with accommodation/tenancy.

(Australian Association of Social Workers, 2016)

> The social work profession is committed to maximising the wellbeing of individuals, families, groups, communities and society. We consider that individual and societal wellbeing is underpinned by socially inclusive communities that emphasise principles of social justice and respect for human dignity and human rights. These values are in complete accord with the disability advocacy movement and the United Nations Convention on the Rights of Persons with Disabilities.
>
> (Australian Association of Social Workers, 2016)

Social workers are actively involved in the disability sector within a number of fields of practice, including: capacity building, community development and engagement, disability services (NGO and government), advocacy services, services for Aboriginal and Torres Strait Islander peoples, health and rehabilitation services, mental health services, child protection, homelessness support, criminal justice services, and educational services. Disability is a cross-sectoral issue but the complexity of the service system; this makes successful navigation difficult for people with disability (Productivity Commission 2017; Madden et al., 2014). Further, the ongoing impacts of the COVID-19 pandemic on people with disability across the lifespan require careful examination and potential policy and service shifts (Yates et al., 2020).

Careful attention to power is required with consideration of what role the social worker can play. The priority must be empowerment of people with disability to make informed choices and decisions about their lives; respecting how they view, understand and embody their disability. Other skill sets identified by the Australian Association of Social Workers (2016) include:

- Capacity building: community engagement, collaboration, consultation, education, awareness raising, and community development.
- Case management: navigation of complex service systems, services brokerage, individualised planning and advocacy, support coordination and referrals.
- Counselling and group work.
- Therapeutic interventions.
- Mediation: conflict resolution and crisis work.
- Policy and program development: monitoring, assessment and evaluation that feeds into modification and redesign.

All the above skills sets should be utilised to ensure privileging of both the voice and agency of people with disability. Critical social workers should embrace co-design that builds upon person-centred and participatory design.

Co-design shares features with collaborative participatory design but the focus is clearly on the person with disability being engaged from the very beginning of any process through to the very end. There is meaningful and respectful engagement throughout the entire process that enables and supports the person with disability to be in the driver's seat (Blomkamp, 2018). Blomkamp (2018) posits that co-design generates innovative ideas, makes sure citizen needs are captured in services provided, and improves responsiveness, fosters cooperation and achieves support for changes required.

Conclusion

Disability represents the larger and more complex interaction between an individual with impairment and the structures and processes of society (Australian Association of Social Workers, 2016). It is imperative that social workers acknowledge that it is not physical, cognitive or sensory impairments that cause disability, but rather the way in which societies fail to accommodate diversity and difference that is an ordinary part of the human condition. Critical social workers should heed advice from Deleuze who argued that disability is best understood as a context-specific articulation of omnipresent difference (Cockayne et al., 2017).

The social work profession embraces human rights, social justice, full citizenship and self-autonomy. Practitioners can work closely with individuals and their families to co-operatively and collaboratively assess needs, articulate and co-develop goals; and, enable people with disability to develop and implement strategies to achieve their desired goals and acquire the skills and knowledge needed to live a quality life in the community. Social workers undertake anti-oppressive practice, so they stand beside people with disability and support them in their efforts for required changes. They may negotiate with express consent on behalf of people with disability and their families; linking with staff and professionals in government and non-government sectors (Australian Association of Social Workers, 2016, 2020). Most importantly, critical social workers bridge the micro/meso and the macro by advocating for systemic changes in the broad socio-political fabric of society to enable people with disability to enjoy voice and agency and most importantly, full citizenship. Regardless of where they work or what roles they undertake, critical social workers must ensure that the needs of people with disability are prioritised and ensure their agency, voice and full participation in society is respected and the key driver of changes required.

Key Website Resources

Australian Association of Social Workers (2016). Scope of Social Work Practice Social Work in Disability (www.aasw.asn.au/document/item/8665UNCRPD).

World Health Organization and the World Bank (2011). World Report on Disability (www.who.int/disabilities/world_report/2011/en).

References

Australian Association of Social Workers. (2016). *Scope of Social Work Practice Social Work in Disability*, Canberra: Australian Association of Social Workers.

Australian Association of Social Workers. (2020). *Code of Ethics*, Melbourne: Australian Association of Social Workers.

Australian Bureau of Statistics. (2019). *Disability, Ageing and Carers, Australia: Summary of findings, 2018*, ABS cat. no. 4430.0, Canberra: Australian Bureau of Statistics.

Australian Institute of Health and Welfare. (2020). *People with Disability in Australia 2020: in brief*, Cat. no. DIS 77, Canberra: Australian Institute of Health and Welfare.

Barnes, C. (2010). A brief history of discrimination and disabled people, in L. Davis. (ed.), *Browne Disability Studies Readers*, Routledge.

Bigby, C. & Frawley, P. (2010). *Social Work Practice and Intellectual Disability*, Palgrave Macmillan.

Bishop, J., & Sunderland, N. (2013). Living with the label 'disability': personal narrative as a resource for responsive and informed practice in biomedicine and bioethics. *Narrative Inquiry in Bioethics*, 3(3), 183–186.

Blomkamp, E. (2018). The Promise of Co-Design for Public Policy, *Australian Journal of Public Administration*, 77(4), 729–743.

Brown, L. (2010), Stigma: An enigma demystified, in L. Davis. (ed.), *Browne Disability Studies Readers*, Routledge.

Buckmaster, L. (2016). *The National Disability Insurance Scheme: A Quick Guide*, Parliament of Australia.

Burns, N. (2017). The human right to health: exploring disability, migration and health. *Disability and Society*, 32(10), 1463–1484.

Carney, T., Then, S., Bigby, C., et al., (2019) National Disability Insurance Scheme plan decision-making: Or when tailor-made case planning met Taylorism and the algorithms. *Melbourne University Law Review*, 42(3), 1–31.

Charlton, J. (2000). *Nothing About Us Without Us: Disability Oppression and Empowerment*, University of California Press.

Chenoweth, L. (2017). Disability, in K. Ellem, W. Chui & J. Wilson (eds), *Social Work and Human Services Best Practice*, 2nd edition, Federation Press.

Chenoweth, L. (2018). *A Brief History of the Disability Services Sector in Australia*, Life Without Barriers.

Chouinard, V., Hall, E., & Wilton, R. (2016). Introduction: Towards enabling geographies, in V. Chouinard, E. Hall and R. Wilson (eds), *Towards Enabling Geographies: 'Disabled' Bodies and Minds in Society and Space*, Routledge.

Cockayne, D., Ruez, D., & Secor, A. (2017). Between ontology and representation: Locating Gilles Deleuze's 'difference-in-itself ' in and for geographical thought, *Progress in Human Geography*, 41(5), 580–599.

Connell, R. (2011) Southern bodies and disability: re-thinking concepts, *Third World Quarterly*, 32 (8), 1369–1381.

Crawford, R., (1980). Healthism and the medicalization of everyday life, *International Journal of Health Sciences*, 10(3):365–388.

Deleuze, G. [1968] (1994) *Difference and Repetition* (translated by P. Patton), Columbia University.

Deleuze, G. (1997). *Essays Critical and Clinical* (translated by D. W. Smith and M. A. Greco), Minneapolis, MN: University of Minnesota Press.

Davis, L. (2010). Constructing normalcy, in L. Davis. (ed.), *Browne Disability Studies Readers*, Routledge.

Degener, T. (2016). Disability in a human rights context. *Laws*, 5(3), 35.

Devine. A., Dickinson, H., Brophy, L. et al., (2019). 'I don't think they trust the choices I will make': Narrative analysis of choice and control for people with psychosocial disability within reform of the Australian Disability Employment Services program, *Public Management Review*, 23(1), 10–30.

Grech, S., & Soldatic, K. (2016). *Disability in the Global South: The Critical Handbook*, Springer.

Harris, B. (2014). The first mental asylums for people with intellectual disabilities, available at developmental disabilities, retrieved from http://ezinearticles.com/?The-First-Mental-Asylums-for-People-With-Intellectual-Disabilities&id=8811115.

Heneker, K.J., Zizzo, G., Awata, M., & Goodwin-Smith, I. (2017). *Engaging Culturally and Linguistically Diverse Communities in the National Disability Insurance Scheme*, Australian Centre for Community Services Research, Flinders University, Adelaide.

Horshell, C. (2020). Problematising disability: A critical policy analysis of the Australian National Disability Insurance scheme, *Australian Social Work*, online ahead of print.

Katsui, H. & Swartz, L. (2021). Research methods and practices of doing disability studies in the Global South. *Scandinavian Journal of Disability Research*, 23(1), 204–206.

Kendrick, M., Ward, M., & Chenoweth, L. (2017). Australia's national disability insurance scheme: looking back to shape the future, *Disability and Society*, 32(9), 1333–1350.

King, J., Edwards, N., Correa-Velez, I., *et al.*, (2016) Disadvantage and disability: Experiences of people from refugee backgrounds with disability living in Australia, *Disability and the Global South*, 3(1), 843–864.

Krnjacki, L., Priest, N., Aitken, Z., *et al.*, (2018). Disability-based discrimination and health: findings from an Australian-based population study, *Australia and New Zealand Journal of Public Health*, 42(2), 172–174.

Lawson, A. & Beckett, A. (2021). The social and human rights models of disability: towards a complementarity thesis, *International Journal of Human Rights*, 25(2), 348–379.

Lemay, R. (1995). Normalization and social role valorisation, in A. Dell Orto and R. Marinelli (eds), *Encyclopedia of Disability and Rehabilitation*, 515–521, Simon and Schuster Macmillan.

Leshota, P. & Sefotho, M. (2020). Being differently abled: Disability through the lens of hierarchy of binaries and Bitso-lebe-ke Seromo, *African Journal of Disability*, 1(9), a643.

Linton, S (2010). Reassigning meaning, in L. Davis (ed.), *The Disability Studies Reader*, 223–236, Routledge.

Madden, R., Fortune, N., Collings, S., *et al.*, (2014). *Cross-Sector Service Coordination for People with High and Complex Needs Harnessing Existing Evidenced and Knowledge*, Centre for Disability Research and Policy, University of Sydney.

Munyi, C. (2012). Past and present perceptions towards disability: A historical perspective, *Disability Studies Quarterly*, 32(2).

National Ethnic Disability Alliance. (2019). *Barriers and Exclusions: The Support Needs of Newly Arrived Refugees with a Disability*, National Ethnic Disability Alliance.

O'Brien, J. (2010). *The Production of Reality: Essays and Readings on Social Interaction*, Sage.

Oliver, M. (1990). The social construction of the disability problem, in *The Politics of Disablement. Critical Texts in Social Work and the Welfare State*, Palgrave.

Olkin, R., Hayward, H., Abbene, M., & VanHeel, G. (2019) The experiences of microaggressions against women with visible and invisible disabilities, *Journal of Social Issues*, 75(3), 757–785.

Olney, S., & Dickinson, H. (2019). Australia's new National Disability Insurance Scheme: Implications for policy and practice, *Policy Design and Practice*, 2(3).

Overboe J. (2012) Theory, impairment and impersonal singularities: Deleuze, Guattari and Agamben, in D. Goodley, B. Hughes & L. Davis (eds), *Disability and Social Theory*, Palgrave Macmillan.

Pelleboer-Gunnink, H., van Weeghel, J., & Embregts, P. (2021). Public stigmatisation of people with intellectual disabilities: a mixed-method population survey into stereotypes and their relationship with familiarity and discrimination, *Disability and Rehabilitation*, 43(4):489–497.

Pilgrim, D., & Tomasini, F. (2012). On being unreasonable in modern society: Are mental health problems special, *Disability and Society*, 27(5), 631–646.

Productivity Commission (2017). National Disability Insurance Scheme (NDIS) costs, retrieved from www.pc.gov.au/inquiries/completed/ndis-costs/report.

Refugee Council of Australia. (2016). Humanitarian arrivals with disability: Discussion paper, retrieved from www.refugeecouncil.org.au.

Sakellariou, D., & Rotarou, E. (2017). The effects of neoliberal policies on access to healthcare for people with disabilities. *International Journal for Equity in Health*, 16(1), 199.

Slade, M. & Longden, E. (2015). Empirical evidence about recovery and mental health, *BMC Psychiatry*, 15(285).

Swartz, L. (2019). Disability and citizenship in the Global South in a post-truth era, in B. Watermeyer, J. McKenzie & L. Swartz (eds) 2019, *The Palgrave Handbook of Disability and Citizenship in the Global South*, 57–65, Palgrave Macmillan.

Temple, J., Kelaher, M. & Williams, R. (2018). Discrimination and avoidance due to disability in Australia: evidence from a national cross-sectional survey. *BMC Public Health*, 18, 1347.

Thill, C. (2019). Listening for intersectionality: How disabled persons' organisations have improved recognition of difference in Australia's National Disability Insurance Scheme, in O. Hankivsky & J. Jordan-Zachery (eds), *The Palgrave Handbook of Intersectionality in Public Policy. The Politics of Intersectionality*, Palgrave Macmillan.

Topor, A., Borg, M., Di Girolamo, S., *et al.* (2011). Not just an individual journey: social aspects of recovery, *International Journal of Social Psychiatry*, 57(1), 90–99.

United Nations. (2006). Convention on the rights of persons with disabilities, retrieved from www.ohchr.org/EN/HRBodies/CRPD/Pages/ConventionRightsPersonsWithDisabilities.aspx.

Velarde, R. (2018). Indigenous perspectives of disability, *Disability Studies Quarterly*, 38(4).

Wells, R., Murad, M., Higgins, M., et.al., (2021). Exploring the intersection of human rights, health, disability and refugee status: an arts-based approach, *Australian Journal of Human Rights*, 26(3), 387–404.

WHO & World Bank. (2011). World report on disability, retrieved from www.who.int/disabilities/world_report/2011/en

Yates, S., Dickinson, H., Smith, C., & Tani, M. (2020). Flexibility in individual funding schemes: How well did Australia's National Disability Insurance Scheme support remote learning for students with disability during COVID-19? *Social Policy & Administration*, 55(5), 906–920.

Part III

Reform Agendas

11 Responding to Suicidal Distress in Social Work Practice

Challenges and Opportunities

Emma Tseris and Charlotte Finlayson

Introduction

In this chapter, we explore social work practices in response to people experiencing suicidal thoughts, feelings, and behaviours. Although suicidal distress is a highly stigmatised experience, having thoughts of death or wanting to die at some point across the life course is a relatively common occurrence, particularly for people who have experienced significant adversity and injustice (Hochhauser et al., 2020). It is important that social workers develop skills in responding to suicidal distress, both at a micro-level in responding to individuals experiencing suicidal thoughts and feelings, as well as at a macro-level, in addressing the social determinants of suicide.

As we commence this chapter, we are aware that the invitation to consider suicidal distress may prompt an array of emotions, including fear, sadness, and confusion. Social workers may have diverse reactions in their work with people experiencing suicidal thoughts and feelings, including concerns about not knowing the right thing to say, or the adverse consequences of doing or saying the wrong thing. Such concerns are understandable, as social work practice occurs within broader community contexts in which long-standing societal taboos, prejudices and myths about suicide have not yet been adequately challenged and reconceptualised (Webb, 2010). Nevertheless, social work has many important contributions to make in both responding to suicidal distress and in suicide prevention.

In this chapter, we critically examine the biomedical paradigm of suicidal distress, which shapes the majority of mental health service responses to suicide within the contemporary Australian context. We explore some themes that are often missing from discussions about mental health practice relating to suicidal distress, namely:

- the relevance of social justice frameworks;
- the importance of broadening our practice beyond risk assessments; and
- the value of meaning-making and sitting with uncertainty.

In doing so, we hope to demonstrate the need for holistic understandings of suicidal distress that are informed by first-person perspectives of 'experts-by-experience', that is, people who have direct experiences of suicidal thoughts and feelings. In order to improve responses to suicidal distress, it is vital that social workers address the historical and ongoing marginalisation of experiential knowledge within mental health services, research, and policy contexts.

DOI: 10.4324/9781003330745-14

Dominant Frameworks for Understanding Suicidality

Biomedical Framework

Contemporary mental health services in Australia and in many other countries are predominantly informed by biomedical perspectives on mental distress. The biomedical paradigm situates human experiences of distress as an 'illness'. As the focus of medicalised interventions is on resolving 'dysfunctions' within individuals, psychiatric diagnoses and medication are offered as a primary response (Morley & Stenhouse, 2021). Yet, evidence for the notion that emotional distress has its origins in bio-genetic factors is faltering (Read & Harper, 2020). These approaches have been critiqued for masking the role of social oppressions and adverse life events, and relying on subjective judgements about what are 'normal' and 'abnormal' human behaviours and experiences (Allsopp et al., 2019).

The biomedical paradigm largely discounts and excludes the perspectives of people who have themselves experienced suicidal distress. This exclusion is based upon the premise that types of knowledge have greater legitimacy and value than others. In the biomedical approach professional and medical 'expertise' is privileged, while knowledge gained through lived experience is seen as less valuable or important (Webb, 2010).

As a result of de-valuing experiential knowledge services fail to allocate resources in ways that respond to the contexts and needs of people experiencing suicidal distress. For example, there are higher rates of suicide within Aboriginal and Torres Strait Islander communities compared to the non-Indigenous population. However, few mental health services are genuinely led by Aboriginal and Torres Strait Islander communities or underpinned by First Nations knowledges of social and emotional wellbeing. The failure to engage with lived experience expertise often leads to culturally inappropriate services that do not address the impacts of colonisation and intergenerational trauma, thus offering a narrow and de-contextualised view of suicidal distress (Dudgeon et al., 2017). This means that he allocation of resources and approaches may reflect pre-determined professional and organisational agendas rather than the needs of people and communities.

Risk-Oriented Framework

Risk assessments are commonly utilised screening tools when working with people experiencing suicidal distress. Risk assessment tools are based upon the assumption that it is possible to make predictions about the likelihood that a person will end their own life by collecting demographic information and asking a series of questions about suicidal thoughts and behaviours (Large et al., 2017). The outcomes of risk assessments are commonly used to determine who is eligible for or excluded from services and what kinds of services are needed. In Australia, and in many other countries, mental health legislation enables people to be treated without consent if they are assessed to be at significant risk to themselves or others. This means that people who are assessed as being at high risk of suicide may be detained and treated involuntarily in hospital.

Limitations of Biomedical and Risk-Oriented Frameworks

Although biomedical and risk-oriented frameworks are the predominant approaches to suicidal distress used in the Australian mental health context, there is limited evidence demonstrating their efficacy. Despite considerable investment in programmes and services, rates of suicide in Australia have remained relatively static (Bastiampillai et al., 2020). Evidence supporting the use of psychotropic medications for suicidal distress is mixed (Jobes, 2017). Involuntary treatment, including hospitalisation, can be traumatising and lead to increased distress. Furthermore, hospitalisation for mental distress is associated with increased risk of suicide post-discharge (Jobes, 2017).

The usefulness of risk assessment tools is also questionable. Meta-analyses of studies on risk assessments demonstrate they are not able to accurately predict who will attempt to act on their suicidal distress (Large et al., 2017). A risk-oriented framework can also have adverse implications for people who are assessed as 'low risk', who may be turned away from services despite voicing distress and requesting support (National Suicide Prevention Taskforce, 2020).

Biomedical and risk-oriented frameworks are shaped by neoliberal discourses, which emphasise individual responsibility for health, locating risk and illness within individuals, while concealing the impacts of social inequalities. By viewing people who are experiencing suicidal primarily through a medical lens, the effects of poverty, violence and other social oppressions on the development of suicidal distress are rendered invisible (Tseris, 2017). A focus on assessing suicide risk can lead to ignoring other kinds of risks in people's lives, for example, housing precarity or racism. This means that people can receive mental health treatment without having the underlying social inequality behind their distress adequately explored or addressed.

The popularity of biomedical and risk-oriented frameworks to suicidality occurs in the context of organisational structures that are risk-averse and concerned with protecting the reputation of organisations and avoiding the scrutiny of managers, the media and the public (Robertson & Collinson, 2011). Unfortunately, this focus can re-direct practice away from meeting the needs of clients towards meeting organisational priorities (Davidson et al., 2016). The dominance of risk assessment tools in the context of responding to suicidal distress can also be understood as related to professionals seeking reassurance and a sense of certainty when engaging with people experiencing suicidal distress, which can be confronting work (Ball & Ritchie, 2020). It is therefore important for mental health workers to acknowledge that it is not possible to reach a place of absolute certainty regarding complex human experiences, and to become more comfortable with sitting with uncertainty and 'not knowing' within mental health practice.

Reflection: The Importance of Humility and Curiosity

> Suicidal feelings are not the same as giving up on life. Suicidal feelings often express a powerful and overwhelming need for a different life.
>
> (Hall, 2013)

Paying attention to first-person accounts of suicidal distress can transform social work practice. As a result of engaging with the mental health consumer/survivor/service user movement, I have learnt more about the invalidating experience of suicide risk assessments and the limitations of biological accounts of mental distress. This has influenced me to reconceptualise my role away from notions of professional 'expertise' towards notions of curiosity and collaboration. I have come to realise that asking a series of questions about suicidal intent and planning often shuts down a much more important conversation about the reasons that a person has become distressed in the first place. Risk assessment tools provide mental health workers with comfort through providing a pre-determined list of questions and the promise of certainty. Nevertheless, human experience is complex, and certainty is therefore an unhelpful aspiration to bring to mental health practice. Over time, I have developed more confidence in 'sitting with' distress, although this is an ongoing process of learning. Rather than being afraid of discussing suicidal thoughts and feelings, I have developed gratitude for the courage that people show in disclosing their experiences and trusting me with their stories. This re-orientation of my role allows me to do more effective listening that is less preoccupied by a pre-determined agenda, and to recognise the deep knowledge that people have about their own lives.

Reflection Questions

1 What opportunities have you had to engage with first-person accounts of suicidal distress, and are you interested to learn more from 'experts-by-experience'? (See 'Key Website Resources' at end of chapter.)
2 What might be some organisational challenges in critiquing biomedical accounts of suicidality and developing practices that are informed by lived experience? What strategies might be useful in negotiating these challenges?

A Social Justice Lens

Analysing Social Contexts

A social justice lens on suicide offers a valuable alternative to biomedical understandings. Rather than situating suicidal distress as evidence of 'illness', a social justice perspective is interested in how suicidal thoughts and feelings can often be linked to situations of social inequality (Hochhauser et al., 2020). A social justice approach to understanding suicide therefore aims to highlight the social and institutional conditions that often give rise to distress. This is demonstrated by the unfair burden of suicidal distress experienced by people in oppressed and marginalised communities (Button, 2016). A social justice approach therefore frames suicide as a socio-political issue, requiring social change and policy responses that are not simply about improving mental health services, but about creating more equitable and inclusive societies. From a social justice perspective, the impacts of colonisation, homophobia and transphobia, ableism, racism, rurality, poverty and homelessness, among many other social contexts and oppressions, are important to consider in understanding why people from some groups and communities are more likely to die by suicide.

The impacts of gender inequality on suicidal distress is a pertinent social context to explore. While patriarchal societies position men as superior and dominant, rigid notions of masculinity are double-edged and can encourage men to be stoic in response to adversity, leading to isolation, self-reliance through distress, and a reluctance to seek help (River & Flood, 2021). Gendered stressors and expectations exert significant power over women's lives as well. While men are more likely to die by suicide in comparison to women, women attempt suicide more frequently than men (Webb, 2010). Domestic violence, sexism within workplaces and communities, and unequal caring responsibilities can place enormous pressures on women, which are relevant factors to consider when exploring the origins of women's suicidal thoughts and feelings (Piper & Stevenson, 2019). The impacts of patriarchal social relations are also relevant to explore when considering suicidal distress among people with trans* or non-binary gender identities. For example, assumptions about a fixed gender binary, which lead to exclusion and discrimination against people who do not perform stereotypical gender roles, are important to consider in understanding the social contexts that may sit behind suicidal distress experienced by gender diverse people (Hunt et al., 2020).

It is important to remember that suicidal distress is a complex and multifaceted experience, which is usually not reducible to a single cause. For this reason, an intersectional lens can be helpful in exploring multiple social injustices and their effects on mental health. For example, gender inequality might intersect with other social oppressions, such as racism or poverty, to further contribute to suicidal distress.

A Narrative Approach

In addition to the need for policy responses to address the social determinants of suicidal distress, a social justice approach has implications for social work practice at a micro-level, including within frontline mental health practice settings. Through a social justice lens, people experiencing suicidal distress can be viewed as responding in meaningful and understandable ways to social suffering and adverse environments, rather than as having 'irrational' thoughts, feelings or behaviours (Ball & Ritchie, 2020). This means people experiencing suicidal distress can be positioned as experts of their own lives, with valuable ideas about how to navigate suicidal distress. In this context, mental health workers can offer a collaborative approach by taking the position of bearing witness to people's narratives and recognising injustices, rather than as detached 'professional experts'.

While it is sometimes assumed that asking a person about suicide may increase suicidal distress, research evidence suggests that asking about suicide can have significant benefits, including reducing suicidal thoughts and behaviours (Stritzke & Page, 2020). Through listening to people's stories, it is possible to explore the strengths that people experiencing suicidal thoughts and feelings have developed over time (Newman, 2016). This exploration can uncover powerful counter-narratives to a biomedical and risk-focused approach, which tends to focus on deficits. Although risk assessments commonly include questions about protective factors, such questions are normally asked in order to contribute towards a calculation of the likelihood of risk. A narrative approach to exploring a person's strengths and supports may allow for less obvious skills, knowledge, and coping strategies to be discussed, which might otherwise go unnoticed by workers (Newman, 2016). This may avoid mental health workers unhelpfully imposing coping strategies onto a person that may not be relevant to a person's context. A collaborative and exploratory approach can lead to a more meaningful discussion by engaging with what people have already been doing to resist oppression and manage suicidal distress.

In addition, a narrative-focused rather than risk-focused approach can be extremely beneficial to developing rapport because it demonstrates care and interest in a person's life. Importantly, a rigid assessment approach to suicidal distress can lead to people answering questions in particular ways, due to fear about the consequences of disclosure (for example, due to fear they will be transported to hospital by police). It has also been noted that an approach to suicidal distress that is focused upon assessing and intervening in response to risk often fails to engage with questions relating to quality of life and addressing the distressing aspects of people's lives that have led to the suicidal distress occurring. A narrative approach can offer a more hopeful response, because it includes an interest not only relating to suicide prevention but also to working collaboratively with clients in order to become 're-engaged with a life worth living' (Stritzke & Page, 2020, p. 3).

Skills for Responding to Suicidal Thoughts and Feelings

Exploring Meaning

Exploring the meaning of suicidality enables social workers to better understand the diverse meanings that suicidal distress can have in people's lives. Rather than making assumptions, a commitment to meaning-making in partnership with people experiencing suicidal distress can reveal new opportunities to address the social drivers of distress. As noted by Will Hall (2013):

> Listen to someone who is suicidal and you often hear a need for change so important, so indispensable, that they would rather die than go on living without the change … Help comes when the person identifies the change they want and starts to believe it can actually happen.

Therefore, through engaging with the details of suicidal distress, rather than a tick-box approach to asking questions about risk, we are likely to develop a much more comprehensive understanding of a person's experiences and environment. This need not involve 'digging' for information, but rather, collaboratively exploring meaning and also being comfortable with using silence to make space for reflection about painful emotions. By taking the time to explore the meaning of suicidal distress, we are not only more likely to come to a detailed and nuanced understanding of a person's experiences, but also a more in-depth understanding of the kinds of supports and responses that might be helpful. By demonstrating a willingness to talk about the suicidal thoughts, rather than treating them as taboo or simply as risks to be managed, people experiencing suicidal distress can feel more supported and affirmed (Newman, 2016).

Advocacy

Although recognising the connections between social injustice and suicidal distress is helpful and validating, it is also important that social workers provide practical support and resources, wherever possible, to respond to injustices and alleviate social suffering. This work involves moving beyond a narrow mental health treatment response in order to address the material realities of people's lives, for example, engaging in advocacy relating to housing precarity or providing practical assistance for women experiencing domestic violence. Social workers can further support clients to navigate highly fragmented services and siloed referral systems that address one issue at a time rather than a person as a whole (National Suicide Prevention Taskforce, 2020).

Social work advocacy is also required within multidisciplinary teams, in order to convey the relevance of social justice perspectives on suicidal distress and the necessity of addressing the social needs of clients (Morley & Stenhouse, 2021). This means questioning a short-term, crisis-driven approach to mental health, which can lead to a vicious cycle whereby people repeatedly access services when highly distressed, with no access to ongoing support to prevent crisis (National Suicide Prevention Taskforce, 2020). Further, it is vital that social workers demonstrate allyship with peer workers within the multidisciplinary team environment, challenging the marginalisation of peer worker perspectives that can occur due to the dominance of biomedical understandings, and advocating for the importance of lived experience expertise in shaping responses to suicidal distress.

Supporting Ourselves in the Work

Finding ways to sustain ourselves as we engage in the complex and challenging work of responding to suicidal distress is another key skill. For social workers new to the field, it may be surprising to note that listening to the stories of people expressing suicidal distress is often not the most significant challenge of working within mental health contexts. Many mental health workers find that listening to people sharing their stories is highly meaningful and rewarding work, and this is especially the case when we focus on the ways in which people have resisted oppression and injustices (Morgan et al., 2019). Major stressors can, however, arise in navigating organisational constraints that are highly risk-averse and that limit the possibilities for utilising a social justice lens. Ideas about self-care that involve individual tasks, such as walking or taking breaks, while useful, can leave workers with an ongoing sense of isolation and without the support that they need to continue to advocate within biomedical environments. Seeking connection with like-minded colleagues who can provide solidarity, and engaging in collective action to address the social determinants of distress is often an invaluable strategy for sustaining ourselves in this work (Reynolds, 2020).

Reflection: Rhiannon's Story

Rhiannon is a 27-year-old Wiradjuri woman living in rural NSW. She is a mother of four children (ages 2, 4, 8 and 10). She also works part-time in a local newsagent. She currently has a supportive mother and partner, however her partner has recently lost his job on one of the local farms, as the farm manager was unable to keep on workers due to the impact of several years of drought. There is also an AVO against her previous partner. Rhiannon uses cannabis recreationally on weekends. She has been referred to your service (the local community mental health team) by the local sexual assault counsellor after she told her counsellor that she had been thinking about taking an intentional overdose on her prescription anti-depressants.

Reflection Questions

1. How would you, as a social worker, approach contacting Rhiannon to arrange an initial appointment? What might you need to take into account in order to do this in a culturally sensitive manner?
2. What do you think might be some important factors to take into account in understanding Rhiannon's story?
3. How could you engage with Rhiannon's protective factors and current supports?
4. How might you advocate for a social justice approach, within the context of a biomedically-oriented multidisciplinary team?
5. What strategies might you draw upon to sustain yourself in this work?

The Role of Prevention

Within the biomedical model 'suicide prevention' is often understood narrowly as a mental health service response to a person who is already experiencing suicidal thoughts and feelings, rather than addressing the social determinants of mental health and creating communities that foster wellbeing. This limited view on suicide prevention reflects the biomedical model of mental health, which focuses on providing 'treatment' once distress has already arisen, without linking emotional suffering to its socio-political roots. A social justice view, which acknowledges the social determinants of suicidal distress, can broaden understandings of the role of social workers.

Consequently, social workers need not see the role of responding to suicide as occurring only in frontline mental health services, but also in an array of other roles that involve addressing unjust social conditions that can lead to suicidal distress. For example, Aboriginal and Torres Strait Islander Elders have outlined the hopelessness and isolation that can arise from a lack of cultural education for First Nations young people, thus demonstrating the importance of connection to culture, community, country, and language as a response to youth suicide (Dudgeon et al., 2017). Through paying attention to these 'bigger picture' components, many opportunities for prevention work, including systemic advocacy and community development, become visible. This means that social workers can be involved not only through direct mental health practice in responding to suicidal thoughts and feelings, but also in addressing the 'upstream' factors of suicidal distress, including colonisation, violence, and social disadvantage (Karban, 2017).

Future Directions

Reducing suicide rates and responding more effectively to suicidal distress has become a priority in Australian health policy. For example, in the 2021–2022 national budget the Commonwealth government committed an additional $2.3 billion to mental health and suicide prevention. While this prioritisation and funding is encouraging, social workers must also bring a critical lens to exploring how suicidal distress is being understood, whether a social justice lens is being used, and the extent to which opportunities for meaningful involvement are being offered to people with first-hand experiences of suicidal thoughts and feelings.

Whilst risk assessment continues to be a mainstream approach to suicide intervention, alternatives to risk assessment are beginning to be explored in some areas. Some scholars argue the discourse of risk has begun to shift in the Global North toward a discourse of 'resilience' (Rose & Lentzos, 2017). This discourse has the potential to be used to re-orient approaches to managing uncertainty away from surveillance and risk management by acknowledging the innate capability of individuals within communities to be able to respond to adversity. However, others have argued resilience discourses conceal social injustice and render individuals responsible for managing the effects of inequalities (Bottrell, 2009).

The idea of resilience has led to increased funding for programmes that emphasise community awareness of suicide. Critics have argued that many of these common training models, such as the mental health first aid courses, are strongly based on the biomedical paradigm and may perpetuate a deficit-focused and symptom-oriented approach (DeFehr, 2016).

A further development is the mainstreaming of peer work and peer advisory groups, which have become one of the pillars of the Fifth National Mental Health and Suicide Prevention Plan (COAG, 2017). For example, peer-led 'Safe Haven' cafes are now open, or in the process of being established, throughout Queensland, New South Wales and Victoria. Based on programmes in the UK, these spaces are intended to provide a non-clinical, trauma-informed alternative to emergency departments, and include the employment of peer workers who have lived experience of suicidal distress. Although this is a promising step, it is still too early to know if such approaches will be effective in shifting the dominant paradigm away from biomedical and risk-focused interventions. In addition, whilst this can be seen as a positive response to long-standing calls for mental health services to incorporate and value the expertise of people with first-hand experiences of mental distress and mental health service provision, it is not yet clear if people with lived experience will be offered meaningful engagement in decision-making processes. As critical mental health scholars and consumer academics have argued, peer engagement should be done in a meaningful and sustained way, not as a 'tick-box' approach (Daya et al., 2020).

Conclusion

In this chapter, we have provided an overview of competing paradigms for understanding and responding to suicidal distress, with an emphasis on the value of a social justice perspective. We hope that this discussion is useful in offering a pathway through the trepidation that might be initially experienced when considering what mental health practice with people experiencing suicidal thoughts and feelings might look like. Social work has much to contribute to responding to suicidal distress, through skills in relationship-building, advocacy, community development, and prevention. The dominance of the biomedical paradigm can result in an over-reliance on pharmaceutical products and hospitalisation to manage distress, while the root causes of suicidal thoughts and feelings remain invisible or under-explored. Through a commitment to engaging with and learning from first-person accounts of suicidal distress, including drawing upon the expertise of peer workers, social workers can move past the limitations of a diagnostic and risk-oriented approach, towards developing practices that are respectful, collaborative, and informed by the complexities of lived experience.

Key Website Resources

Helping the Suicidal Person: Interview with Stacey Freedenthal (https://socialworkpodcast.blogspot.com/2018/04/freedenthal.html). This podcast outlines a narrative approach to understanding suicidal distress, including the limitations of hospitalisation as a response to suicidality.

Living with Suicidal Feelings (https://willhall.net/livingwithsuicidalfeelings). Resources by Will Hall, who is a therapist, host of 'Madness Radio', and person with lived experience of suicidal feelings.

Suicide Narratives (www.humaneclinic.com.au/suicide-narratives). Resources by Humane Clinic in South Australia, premised on the notion that suicidal distress is a response to social suffering rather than an 'illness'.

Thinking about Suicide: Contemplating and Comprehending the Urge to Die (https://thinkingaboutsuicide.org). A companion website for the book *Thinking about Suicide*, by David Webb, who wrote the first PhD on suicide by a person who has attempted suicide.

References

Allsopp, K., Read, J., Corcoran, R. & Kinderman, P. (2019). Heterogeneity in psychiatric diagnostic classification. *Psychiatry research*, 279, 15–22.

Ball, M. & Ritchie, R. (2020). Suicide narratives: Healing through knowing. Retrieved from: www.humaneclinic.com.au/suicide-narratives.

Bastiampillai, T., Allison, S., Looi, J. C., Tavella, A. & Agis, U. (2020). Why are Australia's suicide rates returning to the hundred-year average, despite suicide prevention initiatives? Reframing the problem from the perspective of Durkheim. *Australian & New Zealand Journal of Psychiatry*, 54(1), 12–14.

Bottrell, D. (2009). Understanding 'marginal' perspectives: Towards a social theory of Resilience. *Qualitative Social Work* 8(3), 321–339..

Button, M. E. (2016). Suicide and social justice: Toward a political approach to suicide. *Political research quarterly*, 69(2), 270–280.

COAG. (2017). The fifth national mental health and suicide prevention plan. Retrieved from: www.coaghealthcouncil.gov.au/Portals/0/Fifth%20National%20Mental%20Health%20and%20Suicide%20Prevention%20Plan.pdf.

Davidson, G., Brophy, L. and Campbell, J. (2016). Risk, recovery and capacity: Competing or complementary approaches to mental health social work. *Australian Social Work* 69(2), 158–168.

Daya, I., Hamilton, B. & Roper, C. (2020). Authentic engagement: A conceptual model for welcoming diverse and challenging consumer and survivor views in mental health research, policy, and practice. *International Journal of Mental Health Nursing*, 29(2), 299–311.

DeFehr, J.N. (2016). Inventing mental health first aid: The problem of psychocentrism. *Studies in Social Justice* 10(1), 18–35.

Dudgeon, P., Calma, T. & Holland, C. (2017). The context and causes of the suicide of Indigenous people in Australia. *Journal of Indigenous Wellbeing*, 2(2), 5–15.

Hall, W. (2013). Time for a new understanding of suicidal feelings. Retrieved from: www.madinamerica.com/2013/04/time-for-a-new-understanding-of-suicidal-feelings.

Hochhauser, S., Rao, S., England-Kennedy, E. & Roy, S. (2020). Why social justice matters: a context for suicide prevention efforts. *International Journal for Equity in Health*, 19, 1–8.

Hunt, Q. A., Morrow, Q. J. & McGuire, J. K. (2020). Experiences of suicide in transgender youth: a qualitative, community-based study. *Archives of Suicide Research*, 24(sup2), S340–S355.

Jobes, D. A. (2017). Clinical assessment and treatment of suicidal risk: A critique of contemporary care and CAMS as a possible remedy. *Practice Innovations*, 2(4), 207.

Karban, K. (2017). Developing a health inequalities approach for mental health social work. *British Journal of Social Work*, 47(3), 885–992.

Large, M. M., Ryan, C. J., Carter, G. & Kapur, N. (2017). Can we usefully stratify patients according to suicide risk?. *BMJ*, 359, j4627.

Morgan, H. C., Randall, J., Lyons, A. J., Oliver, S., Saffer, J., Scott, J. M. & Nolte, L. (2019). Pebbles in palms: Counter-practices against despair. *Psychotherapy and Politics International*, 17(1), e1481.

Morley, C. & Stenhouse, K. (2021). Educating for critical social work practice in mental health. *Social Work Education*, 40(1), 80–94.

National Suicide Prevention Taskforce. (2020). Compassion First: Designing our national approach from the lived experience of suicidal behaviour. Retrieved from: www.health.gov.au/resources/publications/national-suicide-prevention-adviser-compassion-first-designing-our-national-approach-from-the-lived-experience-of-suicidal-behaviour.

Newman, D. (2016). How we deal with 'way out thoughts': A living document Ways of talking with young people about suicidal thoughts. *International Journal of Narrative Therapy & Community Work*, 4, 59–66.

Piper, A. & Stevenson, A. (2019). *Gender Violence in Australia: Historical Perspectives*. Monash University Publishing.

Read, J. & Harper, D. J. (2020). The power threat meaning framework: Addressing adversity, challenging prejudice and stigma, and transforming services. *Journal of Constructivist Psychology*, online ahead of print.

Reynolds, V. (2020). Trauma and resistance: 'hang time' and other innovative responses to oppression, violence and suffering. *Journal of Family Therapy*, 42(3), 347–364.

River, J. & Flood, M. (2021). Masculinities, emotions and men's suicide. *Sociology of Health & Illness*, 43(4), 910–927.

Robertson, J. P., & Collinson, C. (2011). Positive risk-taking: Whose risk is it? An exploration in community outreach teams in adult mental health and learning disability services. *Health, Risk & Society*, 13(2), 147–164.

Rose, N., & Lentzos, F. (2017) Making us resilient: Responsible citizens for uncertain times. In S. Trnka and C. Trundle (eds), *Competing Responsibilities*. Duke University Press.

Stritzke, W.G. & Page, A.C. (2020). Suicide is about life. In W. G. Stritzke & A. C. Page (eds), *Alternatives to Suicide* (pp. 3–15). Academic Press.

Tseris, E. (2017). Biomedicine, neoliberalism and the pharmaceuticalisation of society. In B. M. Z. Cohen (ed.), *Routledge International Handbook of Critical Mental Health* (pp. 169–176). Routledge.

Webb, D. (2010). *Thinking about Suicide*. PCCCS Books.

12 Social Work with Aboriginal and Torres Strait Islander People in Health

A Shared Learning, Trauma Informed, Cultural Safety Approach

Melinda Collins, Prue Shanahan, Nicole Watt and Carrie Lethborg

Introduction

Social workers in health settings with Aboriginal and Torres Strait Islander people must ground their practice on an understanding of the history of colonisation, injustice and oppression for this population. The legacy of significant personal and cultural loss for Aboriginal and Torres Strait Islander people continues to impact their lived experiences today through complex trauma, ongoing barriers to accessing health services and ongoing structural racism in many sectors (Carson et al., 2007; Kelly, Dudgeon, Gee & Glaskin, 2009; Holland, Dudgeon & Milroy, 2013; Dudgeon et al., 2014; Parker & Milroy, 2014).

Many Aboriginal and Torres Strait Islander people have been denied access to basic human rights, such as rights to health, housing, employment and education. These are the social determinants of health and they are the conditions in which people are born, grow, live, work and age, and are mostly responsible for health inequalities (World Health Organization, 2020). While understanding this context, social workers must be careful to not assume that trauma is the whole story for this population, as their history is also one of strength that comes from the 'cultural determinants of health', such as connections to culture and Country, that can positively influence outcomes (Brown, 2014). Thus history, social and cultural determinants of health are starting points to understanding Aboriginal and Torres Strait Islander health experiences.

Two-Way Learning

Social work practice should reflect an acknowledgement of these contextual factors, as well as a commitment to shared learning with Aboriginal and Torres Strait Islander colleagues and service users. This 'two-way learning' approach is reflected in the work of Aigner et al. (2014), which suggests that Aboriginal and non-Aboriginal Australians need to build a dialogue, to talk, to work, to lead change. Aigner et al. (2014, p. 74) state that: 'Australia's shared history is dominated by white Australia "doing to" and "doing for" black Australia', and that it is time to acknowledge that we both have the skills, competence and courage to 'do things with' this population. Non-Aboriginal social workers must also consider any unconscious biases and stereotypes they hold given the devastating consequences these can have for Aboriginal and Torres Strait Islander people (Wain et al., 2016).

With the aim of improving the quality of health care for Aboriginal and Torres Strait people,[1] the Social Work Department, Aboriginal staff from the Aboriginal Health Unit

DOI: 10.4324/9781003330745-15

and Mental Health Services at St Vincent's Hospital, Melbourne (SVHM) have used dialogue and collaboration, to, over time, build cultural respect and responsiveness to transform patient care. In this process, non-Aboriginal social workers have adopted the position, with humility and respect, that in relation to Aboriginal health we are learners, not experts. Day to day, through dialogue/'yarning' and learning from each other and by commitment to working together, incremental change and improvements in practice have occurred. The social work team has also been guided by available literature, reports and materials from the Aboriginal health policy domain, which is generated or informed by Aboriginal and Torres Strait Islander communities, organisations and stakeholders.

This collaborative process has resulted in new methods and tools for practice and training. Some of the jointly developed social work and Aboriginal Health tools at SVHM include: a quick resource and discharge checklist and tools to aid joint Aboriginal Hospital Liaison Officer (AHLO) and social work care planning and referral documents. This chapter has been written as a collaboration between Aboriginal and non-Aboriginal staff from St Vincent's Hospital, Melbourne (SVHM) and reflects the model of care developed over time at SVHM and that we hope is helpful for other social workers in the health setting.

Context

The Australian Association of Social Workers (AASW) recognises the many historical injustices that have shaped the lived experience of Aboriginal and Torres Strait Islander people and the still unmet need for reconciliation in this country. In 2004, the AASW published an 'Acknowledgement Statement to Aboriginal and Torres Strait Islander People', which recognised the dispossession and removal, disempowerment and disenfranchisement of Aboriginal and Torres Strait Islander people and the historical actions of non-Aboriginal social workers and others in implementing unjust policies that led to the creation of the Stolen Generation (Australian Association of Social Workers, 2004). These injustices and trans-generational trauma are core reasons why Aboriginal and Torres Strait Islander people remain at greater risk of ill health and reduced wellbeing with a life expectancy of around ten years less than non-Aboriginal Australians (Department of the Prime Minister and Cabinet, 2019).

It is well recognised that Aboriginal and Torres Strait Islander people do not always access mainstream health services even when they need them (Mackean et al., 2020; Barnett & Kendall, 2011). Reasons for this reluctance include services not being person centred or welcoming, fear and mistrust by individuals due to previous experiences that have been culturally unsafe and stories passed down through families of traumatic experiences in such settings (Orr, Frederico & Long, 2021; Gomersall et al., 2017). It is important that social workers know about lived experiences of Aboriginal and Torres Strait Islander people in mainstream health settings.

Learning from Stories of Lived Experience

Nyernila Koories Kila Degaia: Listen Up to Koories Speak about Health (Vickery et al., 2005) and *Lookin' after Our Own: Supporting Aboriginal Families through Hospital Experience* (Clarke et al., 1999) offer poignant examples of such experiences. In 2005, Vickery et al. collated oral histories by Aboriginal people and others about Aboriginal people's experience of mainstream health care.

Vickery et al. (2005) collection of stories compellingly conveys experiences of exclusion, discrimination and segregation. Aboriginal people describe being treated at the back of, or on the verandas of, hospitals (Vickery et al., 2005, pp. 80, 106). One community member shared, 'if there was a public toilet you weren't allowed to use it. In a hospital setting we were segregated from non-Indigenous people, and the mannerisms of doctors, the gentleness and compassion, wasn't there' (Vickery et al., 2005, p. 17). Another said, 'one of the things that sticks out in my memory is when a Koorie went into hospital, regardless of whose kid it was, first thing was it was bathed and deloused and dewormed. This was regardless of whatever it had, you know' (Vickery et al., 2005, p. 92).

Vickery et al. (2005) also described how the costs associated with medication and accessing health care were often difficult for Koorie people to afford and that decisions had to be made between paying for the cost of health care or feeding the family (Vickery et al., 2005, p. 128). Negative experiences led to fear and mistrust. Aboriginal people were often admitted to hospital late or 'on their last legs' (Vickery et al., 2005, p. 56) when they were too acutely ill for treatment to make a difference. Hospitals then became known or associated with death and dying, rather than as a place to for improvements in health. 'A lot of old people got into the lift and never came back. And that lift was sort of seen as a taboo' (Vickery et al., 2015, p. 56).

Other experiences are documented in submissions and evidence provided to the Report of the National Inquiry into the Separation of Aboriginal and Torres Strait Islander Children from their Families (1997), where a common thread strongly suggested that hospitals throughout Australia, over a number of decades, were systematically involved in the removal of Aboriginal children from their loved ones and kin (Clarke et al., 1999, p. 40). The experiences described by these authors are disquieting and sobering and important to read. Given these experiences, disparities in health outcomes and socio-economic disadvantage, we argue that Aboriginal and Torres Strait Islander patients and families should be given a high priority response and support by social work in health services. In a study by Harms et al. (2012) social work practitioners identified practice models that they use in Aboriginal communities to include anti-oppressive crisis intervention; advocacy; solution focussed, single-session or brief intervention; strengths and narrative approaches; and client-centred approaches (Harms et al., 2012, p. 20).

Unique Conceptualisation of Health

Social workers must also understand that Aboriginal and Torres Strait Islander people do not view health just in relation to the physical wellbeing of the individual but the social, emotional and cultural wellbeing of the whole community. In this view, health is based on connections to country, culture, community, family, spirit and physical and mental health (Dudgeon et al., 2014, Gee et al., 2014). While social workers are trained to consider the person in their environment and have a systems approach to understanding the impact of illness, they are still challenged to engage in a narrow medically focused model of both care and funding that can impact the priorities of health care organisations.

The National Strategic Framework for Aboriginal and Torres Strait Islander Mental Health and Social and Emotional Wellbeing 2017–2023 has proposed the incorporation of the Social and Emotional Well-Being (SEWB) Model into health care settings (Gee et al., 2014; Department of the Prime Minister and Cabinet, 2017). Many Aboriginal Community Controlled Health Service (ACCHSs) utilise this model already. At SVHM, the Aboriginal Health Unit introduced the SEWB Model into practice and offer training in its translation into practice, including an 'Aboriginal Social & Emotional Wellbeing Formulation' plan which can be completed and included in a patient's online medical record.

Trauma Informed/Cultural Safety

Given these contextual factors, a trauma informed, culturally safe framework offers an important model for social work to follow when working with Aboriginal and Torres Strait Islander people. This model begins by acknowledging the experience of trauma as a common experience both personally and/or shared through generations for this population (Atkinson, Nelson and Atkinson, 2010). Trauma has an ongoing impact on physical, emotional, and mental health and on engagement to health services (Buckley, Green & Schnurr, 2004). Trauma-informed care further acknowledges the role of health services in re-traumatising people and aims to counter these experiences and offer a strength based, holistic and culturally appropriate approach to service delivery (Substance Abuse and Mental Health Services Administration, 2014).

Safety and Trust

A trauma-informed approach to Aboriginal and Torres Strait Islander health focuses on creating a safe environment that enables trust, choice, collaboration, and empowerment so that healthy relationships with service providers and positive outcomes in their care can occur (Harris & Fallot, 2001; Elliott, Bjelajac, Fallot, Markoff & Reed, 2005; Lethborg et al., 2021). To this end, the previously noted contextual understanding for this population's history and culture informs the importance of safety, respect, and acceptance in the helping relationship, and the establishment of an atmosphere of trust (Elliott et al., 2005). For Aboriginal and Torres Strait Islander people who have not experienced culturally safe health services, trust needs to be earned and demonstrated over time. This approach acknowledges that attending health services can be anxiety provoking and encompasses a heightened awareness of the possibility of trauma. The social worker needs to recognise that the burden is on them to facilitate trust and that this requires a compassionate and respectful way of engaging with the person, their family and their culture.

Social workers should model respectful interpersonal boundaries, language, and use of power so that safe and appropriate limits, and predictability can be set without recreating experiences of oppression (Harris & Fallot, 2001; Elliott et al., 2005). Cultural safety is centred on the subjective experience of the person receiving support and requires the social worker to be responsive to the differing cultural needs of Aboriginal and Torres Strait Islander people whilst being attuned how their own values impact the care provided (Elvidge, Paradies, Aldrich & Holder, 2020). Social workers must be prepared to recognise that they may make mistakes in practice with Aboriginal and Torres Strait Islander people and professional pathways are needed to demonstrate an understanding of the issue and how to correct it.

The helping styles of Aboriginal social workers offer specific insight about how engagement and respect are central to developing a safe relationship with Aboriginal and Torres Strait Islander people in the health context (Harms et al., 2012). Referring to the work of Lynn (2001), this is described as the 'use of self' in the helping context, the importance of spirituality, the use of a holistic approach and 'there is recognition of a cultural difference as a strength, rather than a weakness, as a resource rather than a problem' (Lynn, 2001, p. 6). In aspects of the helping process there are differences in the language and activities of indigenous workers, and the use of self-disclosure in their interventions.

Bennett and Zubrzycki (2003) outline that Aboriginal social workers articulate a different practice reality in which their cultural, personal and professional identities converge. Aboriginal social workers use self-disclosure, such as identifying birthplace and kinship ties, as well as sharing personal stories and life experiences, to enhance the helping relationship and establish credibility with clients (Bennett & Zubrzycki, 2003).

Safety and trust are central to developing genuine engagement with Aboriginal and Torres Strait Islander people whose social and emotional wellbeing results from a network of relationships between individuals, family, kin and community (Department of the Prime Minister and Cabinet, 2017). As such, any social work assessment and intervention must focus on and incorporate the social and emotional wellbeing of Aboriginal patients, their families and communities. The importance of genuine relational engagement in this setting was further described by Bennett et al. (2011) who reported experienced Aboriginal and non-Aboriginal social workers prioritise the development of relationships with their Aboriginal clients and communities which are characterised by reciprocity, the integration and valuing of Aboriginal and Western world-views, and the application of micro skills, such as 'deep listening'/*dadirri* and 'stillness' (Ungunmerr-Baumann, 2002). The authors of this chapter would also like to emphasise narrative approaches in developing safety and trust (White & Epston, 1990) because they remind us to listen to the stories and to allow time and space to sit and have discussions with Aboriginal patients and families in an unhurried way.

Collaboration, Choice, Empowerment

Trauma-informed care aims to develop a shared power relationship to ensure a true alliance in healing, this is important not only because of the inherent power imbalance in the 'helping' relationship between social worker and client but is potentially of greater importance with Aboriginal and Torres Strait Islander people because of historical injustices (Elliott et al., 2005; Fallot & Harris, 2009; Morrison et al., 2019). A trauma-informed approach aims to support the person's own decision making and a sense of control over their own health needs (Fallot & Harris, 2009). This can transform them from a position of powerlessness to a person who directs and owns his or her life decisions and the associated outcomes (Elliott et al., 2005). Green and Baldry (2005) also highlight that, if power differentials are to be truly challenged, Aboriginal and Torres Strait Islander worldviews must be privileged in this approach.

Developing a partnership with the Aboriginal person that is empowering and genuinely centred on their identified needs is central to a trauma informed approach and must include their Aboriginal Health workers, family and community members. Social workers should focus on ways that 'convey respect and compassion, honour self-determination, and enable the rebuilding of healthy interpersonal skills and coping strategies' (Levenson, 2017). This kind of approach offers a powerful setting in which the Aboriginal person can, sometimes for the first time, experience the opportunity to express their needs and to be heard within a mainstream health service. Indeed, a warm, interested, and validating therapeutic alliance is more influential in facilitating positive outcomes than theoretical frameworks, professional strategies or techniques (Wampold, 2001; Duncan, Miller, Wampold & Hubble, 2010).

A collaborative approach also minimises the potential to define Aboriginal and Torres Strait Islander people by a common narrative of 'vulnerability', rather it offers the chance to incorporate a strengths-based focus and respond to the person and their unique experiences (Kezelman & Stavropoulos, 2019). The social worker should also seek to understand the broad implications of the persons health needs, including the impact and resources surrounding the person, their family and community. In most cases, engagement with Aboriginal health services such as Aboriginal Community Controlled Health Service (ACCHSs) is also important. ACCHSs are community driven and operate in metropolitan, regional, rural and remote areas of all states and territories in Australia. These services are of critical importance for referral, planning, assistance and liaison prior to admission or attendance at a tertiary hospital, during the hospital stay and for the provision of continuing care. See the National Aboriginal Community Controlled Health Organisation (NACCHO) website for further information about Aboriginal Community Controlled Health.

In Summary

When working with Aboriginal and Torres Strait Islander people, social workers and AHLOs at SVHM suggest that practitioners:

- Ensure early welcome and timely contact by AHLOs and/or social work with Aboriginal patients and families.
- Let the person tell their story, be patient and listen attentively.
- Be aware of your body language and verbal communication – for example, position in the room, eye contact, tone of voice and use of language.
- Involve the AHLO, patient, family and community in collaborative assessment and planning.
- Dialogue and collaborate to work out what needs to be done and how. At times there will be sensitivities to consider. For example, patients and/or family members may have kinship or community ties with the AHLO, which may add a degree of stress at an emotional level, in terms of expectations and felt pressure.
- Consider what practical supports and material aid Aboriginal and Torres Strait Islander patients and families need and what resources the health service can offer. This may require developing new options.
- Consider the value of joint social work and AHLO documentation processes; for example, if both are involved in interviews, family meetings or case conferences.
- Consider convening complex care review meetings. At SVHM, AHLOs and social workers and invited key staff meet weekly to review Aboriginal and Torres Strait Islander patient complex care issues and consider possible solutions. While this has clear consultation, planning and coordination benefits, the format provides a vibrant opportunity for 'working together/two way learning'.
- Importantly, if you make a mistake – whether it is self-identified or highlighted by an Aboriginal or Torres Strait Islander person - apologise and move forward together.

Reflection: Terry's Story

A Brief Overview

Terry is a 49-year-old single Aboriginal man who lives in a ministry of housing flat in metropolitan Melbourne and receives the disability support pension. He has been diagnosed with lymphoma, a form of blood cancer, during the admission. He has commenced his treatment as inpatient and then will move to outpatient treatment.

Terry finds the hospital environment very challenging as it restricts his freedom and reminds him of past bad experiences. He has left the ward for several hours at a time on a few occasions when he has become distressed and can't tolerate the environment anymore. Terry's distress may present as verbal aggression towards staff leading some staff to label him as a 'difficult patient'.

You have been asked to meet with Terry and complete a social work assessment in light of his cancer diagnosis and reaction to being in hospital.

Social Work Role and Process Considerations

To understand Terry's needs and behaviours, it is essential that the social worker use their expertise to help the team incorporate a trauma informed response (Blue Knot Foundation, 2019). Additionally, given the multifaceted supportive care needs of Aboriginal and Torres Strait Islander people with cancer, appropriate support can only occur when it is co-designed with the patient, their family, AHLOs, the hospital team and community (Lethborg et al., 2021).

1. What could you do to help Terry feel safer in the hospital environment?

Consider:

Engaging with the AHLO as early as possible.
Have the AHLO introduce you to Terry (and family where appropriate) – this provides a way for the AHLO to facilitate the relationship between Aboriginal services, social workers and also other members of the health care team (Bnads et al., 2020).
Be mindful of your body language and your verbal communication.
Observe carefully any signs and symptoms of distress Terry may be displaying – recognise and address these.
Ask Terry how you can help him feel more settled and safe in the hospital. What does he need?

2. How could you use the SEWB model with Terry?

Consider:

Completing a joint assessment(s) with the AHLO – consider a plan whereby you both explore Terry's connection to spirit, spirituality and ancestors and connection to country and culture together.
Be mindful to listen attentively to Terry, do not hurry him, and be present and engaged. Do not follow a set agenda.

With the above considerations, and in discussion and collaboration with Terry, the AHLO, his family, you could devise the following

Aboriginal Social & Emotional Wellbeing Formulation Plan

Connection to spirit, spirituality and ancestors: Terry feels a deep connection to his ancestors and feels that they guide him through life.

Connection to country: Terry is very connected to his home country which he grew up on. COVID lockdowns are difficult for him as he can't return to Country at a time when he most feels he needs to be there to heal.

Connection to culture: Terri is very connected to his culture but is feeling disconnected during COVID as a lot of programmes are not running. He is especially missing the weekly Men's Group.

Connection to community: Terry prefers to use Aboriginal health & community services. Terry is connected to the local Aboriginal community and his local community on Country. He has workers at the Aboriginal Health Service and likes to receive an Aboriginal Hospital Liaison Officer service for cultural support when he is admitted to hospital.

Connection to family and kinship: Terry has 1 sister and 2 brothers, they are members of the Stolen Generations having been removed from their parents' care early in their lives. Both of Terry's parents are deceased. Terry's older sister lives in regional Victoria and is very worried about him. *She is worried how he will get to treatment and what will happen if he becomes sick after treatment. She feels frustrated she cannot help him more but she lives far away. Terry has limited contact with his two younger brothers but wishes he could see them more.*

Connection to mind and emotions: Terry has complex post-traumatic stress disorder from trauma he experienced in his childhood and finds it very difficult to talk about the past. *Terry finished school in Year 8. He has difficulty reading information and finds it hard to take in a lot of information at once. He can become frustrated when he doesn't understand something and he may react by lashing out verbally. He hates being in hospital given some of his past experiences which he finds difficult to talk about.*

Connection to body: *Terry has been diagnosed with cancer. He is worried his treatment will make him feel sick and tired and stop him doing things he enjoys.*

3. How would you help Terry and his family feel empowered and in control with decision making about his health care?

Consider:

Ask Terry how you can help him. What does he need?
Ask Terry if there is anyone else who would like the team to speak to - it could be family, an Elder, members of his community and Aboriginal health and community services.
Ask Terry how it is best to give him information about his illness and treatment. Ensure the treating team are aware of this.
Advocate for Terry within the team - educate them that Terry's reactions are indicators of his fear of being in hospital, feeling frustrated and not understanding his health care at the moment.
Convening a family meeting to keep Terry and his family informed and involved in his care.
Convening a case planning/complex care meeting with hospital and community staff to ensure everyone is aware and addressing Terry's needs – both now and for the duration of his treatment.
Together with the AHLO, introduce Terry to the outpatient clinic and team where he will receive his ongoing treatment.
What other supports/staff can be accessed? e.g. Aboriginal Health Community Services, psycho-oncology team, specialist cancer organisations.

What can be done to support Terry's sister and address her needs?
What practical supports can be arranged (e.g. transport to treatment, financial assistance, ongoing and collaborative Social Work and AHLO involvement throughout Terry's treatment)?

Relevant Guidelines

Social workers need to be aware of formal guidelines and resources for Aboriginal and Torres Strait Islander health care, as these align with policy and practice. Basic knowledge on the following is useful:

- National best practice guidelines for collecting Indigenous health status data sets (Australian Institute of Health and Welfare, 2010). It is mandatory for Australian hospitals to ask every patients 'Are you of Aboriginal or Torres Strait Islander origin?'
- The Australian Association of Social Worker's guideline 'Preparing for culturally responsive and inclusive social work practice in Australia: working with Aboriginal and Torres Strait Islander peoples' (Australian Association of Social Workers, 2016).
- A Reconciliation Action Plan (RAP) is a strategic framework that assists organisations in their efforts to support reconciliation with Aboriginal and Torres Strait Islander peoples - for example, the Australian 'Association of Social Workers Innovate Reconciliation Action Plan July 2020 – June 2022'. Social Workers are encouraged to research their own Organisations' RAP.
- National Safety and Quality in Health Care (NSQHS) 'User Guide for Aboriginal and Torres Strait Islander Health' provides information for health service organisations to help them improve the quality of care and health outcomes for Aboriginal and Torres Strait Islander people based on the National Safety and Quality Health Service Standards.
- Grief and loss are core areas of work for health social workers. Resources on how to work effectively and provide Aboriginal culturally sensitive support where there is sad news or 'sorry business' have been developed by different jurisdictions; for example, Queensland Health (State of Queensland, 2015).

Conclusion

When working with Aboriginal and Torres Strait Islander people, social workers in health care must engage with a shared learning, trauma informed and cultural safety approach. Social workers must have an understanding of Aboriginal and Torres Strait Islander people's history and the social and cultural determinants of health. In possessing this, social workers can begin to understand the lived experience of Aboriginal and Torres Strait Islander people, the barriers faced in accessing mainstream health care in a culturally safe way and begin to address the multifaceted needs of Aboriginal and Torres Strait Islander people through a shared learning approach with Aboriginal health colleagues, patients and communities.

We would like to conclude this chapter with quotes from an AHLO and a social worker on the benefits of shared learning approach:

> The learning really goes both ways. As an AHLO I learn from social workers and I am developing my knowledge and competencies. Working together also means I have stronger connections to other people in the multidisciplinary team. Having a good working relationship is positive because it means better outcomes for patients. You can see this from the way we integrate discharge referrals.
>
> (SVHM AHLO)

> Our collaborative approach contributes to comprehensive psychosocial care by ensuring that the cultural needs of Aboriginal patients are acknowledged and respected. It reinforces the importance of patient centred care and – for me – that cultural awareness develops as we work together.
>
> (SVHM social worker)

Acknowledgement

The authors would like to acknowledge Sonia Posenelli, Toni Mason and Michelle Gallagher Winters, for not only their invaluable leadership and contribution to the previous edition of this chapter, but also for their unwavering commitment to embedding a shared learning model of care between Aboriginal health and social work at SVHM.

Key Website Resources

This list of key websites is not exhaustive but is intended to provide a starting point for further investigation and research.

Aboriginal and Torres Strait Islander Health (Australian Government Department of Health) (www.health.gov.au/health-topics/aboriginal-and-torres-strait-islander-health).

Australian Indigenous HealthInfoNet (https://healthinfonet.ecu.edu.au).

Australian Institute of Aboriginal and Torres Strait Islander Studies (AIATSIS) (https://aiatsis.gov.au).

Closing the Gap: In Partnership (Australian Government) (www.closingthegap.gov.au).

Common Ground (www.commonground.org.au).

Indigenous Australians (AIHW) (www.aihw.gov.au/reports-data/population-groups/indigenous-australians/overview).

The Indigenous Australians' Health Program (IHAP) (Australian Department of Health) (www.health.gov.au/initiatives-and-programs/indigenous-australians-health-programme).

Indigenous.gov.au (Australian Government) (www.indigenous.gov.au).

Lowitja Institute (www.lowitja.org.au).

National Aboriginal Community Controlled Health Organisation (NACCHO) (www.naccho.org.au).

National Indigenous Australians Agency (NIAA) (Australian Government) (www.niaa.gov.au/

Reconciliation Australia (www.reconciliation.org.au).

Understanding Indigenous welfare and wellbeing (Australian Institute of Health and Welfare – AIHW) (www.aihw.gov.au/reports/australias-welfare/understanding-indigenous-welfare-and-wellbeing).

Note

1 In keeping with the (SVHA cultural guidelines title) this chapter will use the term 'Aboriginal and Torres Strait Islander people' when referring to the population known as Indigenous, Aboriginal, Aboriginal and Torres Strait Islander(s); Koori(e), and other titles specific to localities, such as Murri and Nyungah. When the authors of this chapter draw on literature or when the names of policies, services and programs are used, the authors use from those sources. When the term 'Aboriginal' is used in relation to SVHM practice, this is inclusive of Aboriginal and Torres Strait Islander people.

References

Aigner, G., Godwell, C., Martin, J., Paulson, G., Rawnsley, J., Robertson, K., Skelton, L., Varcoe, L. & Yettica-Paulson (2014). *Lost Conversations*. Melbourne: Creative Commons.

Atkinson, J., Nelson, J. & Atkinson, C. (2010). Trauma, transgenerational transfer and effects on community wellbeing. In N. Purdie, P. Dudgeon & R. Walker (eds), *Working Together: Aboriginal and Torres Strait Islander Mental Health and Wellbeing Principles and Practice*, 135–144. Canberra: Australian Government Department of Health and Ageing.

Atkinson, J. (2013). *Trauma-Informed Services and Trauma-Specific Care for Indigenous Australian Children*. Resource sheet no. 21. Produced for the Closing the Gap Clearinghouse. Canberra: Australian Institute of Health and Welfare & Melbourne: Australian Institute of Family Studies.

Australian Association of Social Workers. (2004). Acknowledgement statement to Aboriginal and Torres Strait Islander people. Retrieved from www.aasw.asn.au/document/item/618.

Australian Association of Social Workers. (2016). Preparing for culturally responsive and inclusive social work practice in Australia: working with Aboriginal and Torres Strait Islander peoples – January 2015. Retrieved from www.aasw.asn.au/document/item/7006.

Australian Commission on Safety and Quality in Health Care. (2017). National Safety and Quality Health Service Standards: User guide for Aboriginal and Torres Strait Islander health. Retrieved from www.safetyandquality.gov.au.

Australian Institute of Health and Welfare. (2010). *National Best Practice Guidelines for Collecting Indigenous Status in Health Data Sets*. Cat. no. IHW 29. Canberra: AIHW.

Barnett, L. & Kendall, E. (2011). Culturally appropriate methods for enhancing the participation of Aboriginal Australians in health-promoting programs. *Health Promotion Journal of Australia*, 22(1), 27–32.

Bennett, B. & Zubrzycki, J. (2003). Hearing the stories of Australian Aboriginal and Torres Strait Islander social workers: challenging and educating the system. *Australian Social Work*, 56, 61–70.

Bennett, B., Zubrzycki, J. & Bacon, V. (2011). What do we know? The experiences of social workers working alongside Aboriginal people? *Australian Social Work*, 64(1), 20–37.

Blue Knot Foundation. (2019). Trauma informed care and practice. Retrieved from www.blueknot.org.au/Workers-Practitioners/For-Health-Professionals/Resources-for-Health-Professionals/Trauma-Informed-Care-and-practice.

Bnads, H., Orr, E. & Clements, C.J. (2020). Improving the service to Aboriginal and Torres Strait Islanders through innovative practices between Aboriginal hospital liaison officers and social workers in hospitals in Victoria, Australia. *British Journal of Social Work*, online ahead of print.

Brown, N. (2014). Exploring cultural determinants of health and wellbeing. Retrieved from www.lowitja.org.au/content/Document/PDF/Ngaire-Brown.pdf.

Buckley, T. C., Green, B. L. & Schnurr, P, P. (2004), Trauma, PTSD, and physical health: *PTSD*, 441–465. The Guilford Press.

Carson, B. (2007). *Social Determinants of Indigenous Health*. Crows Nest, NSW: Allen & Unwin.

Clarke, A., Andrews, S. & Austin, N. (1999). *Lookin' After Our Own: Supporting Aboriginal Families through the Hospital Experience*. Melbourne: Aboriginal Family Support Unit – Royal Children's Hospital.

Department of the Prime Minister and Cabinet. (2017). *National Strategic Framework for Aboriginal and Torres Strait Islander Peoples' Mental Health and Social and Emotional Wellbeing 2017–2023*. Canberra: Department of the Prime Minister and Cabinet.

Department of the Prime Minister and Cabinet. (2019). *Closing the Gap*. Canberra: Department of the Prime Minister and Cabinet.

Dudgeon, P., Wright, M., Paradies, Y., Garvey, D. & Walker, I. (2014). Aboriginal social, cultural and historical contexts. In P. Dudgeon, H. Milroy & R. Walker (eds), *Working Together: Aboriginal and Torres Strait Islander Mental Health and Wellbeing Principles and Practice*. Canberra: Office of Aboriginal and Torres Strait Islander Health, Department of Ageing.

Duncan, B. L., Miller, S. D., Wampold, B. E. & Hubble, M. A. (eds). (2010). *The Heart and Soul of Change: Delivering What Works in Therapy* (2nd ed.). American Psychological Association.

Elliott, D. E., Bjelajac, P., Fallot, R. D., Markoff, L. S. & Reed, B. G. (2005), Trauma-informed denied: Principles and implementation of Trauma-informed services for women. *Journal of Community Psychology*, 33(4), 461–477.

Elvidge, E., Paradies, Y., Aldrich, R. & Holder, C. (2020). Cultural safety in hospitals: validating an empirical measurement tool to capture the Aboriginal patient experience. *Australian Health Review*, 44(2), 205–211.

Fallot, R. D. & Harris, M. (2009). *Creating Cultures of Trauma-Informed Care*. Washington, DC: Community Connections.

Gee, G., Dudgeon, P., Schultz, C., Hart, A. & Kelly, K. (2014). *Aboriginal and Torres Strait Islander social and emotional wellbeing*. In P. Dudgeon, H. Milroy & R. Walker (eds), *Working Together: Aboriginal and Torres Strait Islander Mental Health and Wellbeing Principles and Practice*, 55–68. Canberra: Office of Aboriginal and Torres Strait Islander Health, Department of Ageing.

Gomersall, J. S., Gibson, O., Dwyer, J., O'Donnell, K., Stephenson, M., Carter, D., Canuto, K., Munn, Z., Aromataris, E. & Brown A. (2017). What Indigenous Australian clients value about primary health care: a systematic review of qualitative evidence. *Australian and New Zealand Journal of Public Health*, 41(4), 417–423.

Green, S. & Baldry, E. (2005). Building Indigenous Australian social work. *Australian Social Work*, 61(4), 89–402.

Harms, L., Clarke, A., Anderson, I., Whyte, J., Middleton, J. & Sloan, J. (2012). *From Colonisation to Conciliation: An Exploration of Social Work Practice with Aboriginal Populations*. Melbourne: University of Melbourne.

Harris, M. & Fallot, R. D. (eds). (2001). *Using Trauma Theory to Design Service Systems*. Jossey-Bass/Wiley.

Holland, C., Dudgeon, P. & Milroy, H (2013). *The Mental Health and Social and Emotional Wellbeing of Aboriginal and Torres Strait Islander Peoples, Families and Communities*. Canberra: National Mental Health Commission.

Kelly, K., Dudgeon, P., Gee, G. & Glaskin, B. (2009). *Living on the Edge: Social and Emotional Wellbeing and Risk and Protective Factors for Serious Psychological Distress among Aboriginal and Torres Strait Islander People*. Discussion Paper No. 10. Darwin: Cooperative Research Centre for Aboriginal Health.

Kezelman, C. A. &Stavropoulos P. A. (2019). *Practice Guidelines for Clinical Treatment of Complex Trauma*. Blue Knot Foundation.

Lethborg, C., Halatanu, F., Mason, T., Posenelli, S., Cleak, H. & Braddy, L. (2021). Culturally informed, codesigned, supportive care for Aboriginal and Torres Strait Islander people with cancer and their families. *Australian Social Work*, online ahead of print. doi:10.1080/0312407X.2021.1916050.

Levenson J, (2017). Trauma-informed social work practice. *Social Work*, 62(2), 105.

Lynn, R. (2001). Learning from a 'Murri way'. *The British Journal of Social Work*, 31(6), 903–916.

Mackean, T., Withall, E., Dwyer, J. & Wilson, A (2020). Role of Aboriginal Health Workers and Liaison Officers in quality care in the Australian acute care setting a systematic review. *Australian Health Review*, 44, 427–433.

Morrison, A., Rigney, L.I., Hattam, R. & Diplock, A. (2019). Toward an Australian culturally responsive pedagogy: A narrative review of the literature. Retrieved from https://apo.org.au/node/262951.

Orr, E., Frederico, M. & Long, M. (2021). Messages for good practice: Aboriginal hospital liaison officers and hospital social workers. *Australian Social Work*, online ahead of print. doi:10.1080/0312407X.2021.1953552.

Parker, R. & Milroy, H. (2014). Aboriginal and Torres Strait Islander mental health: An overview. In P. Dudgeon, H. Milroy & R. Walker (eds), *Working Together: Aboriginal and Torres Strait Islander Mental Health and Wellbeing Principles and Practice*. Canberra: Office of Aboriginal and Torres Strait Islander Health, Department of Ageing.

State of Queensland. (2015). Sad news, sorry business: guidelines for caring for Aboriginal and Torres Strait Islander people through death and dying (version 2). Retrieved from www.health.qld.gov.au/__data/assets/pdf_file/0023/151736/sorry_business.pdf.

Substance Abuse and Mental Health Services Administration. (2014). *SAMHSA's Concept of Trauma and Guidance for a Trauma-Informed Approach*. Rockville, MD: Substance Abuse and Mental health Services, Administration.

Ungunmerr-Baumann, M. R. (2002). DaddirriL inner deep listening and quiet still awareness. Retrieved from www.dadirri.org.au/wp-content/uploads/2015/03/Dadirri-Inner-Deep-Listening-M-R-Ungunmerr-Bauman-Refl1.pdf.

Vickery, J., Clarke, A, Adams, K. (2005). *Editors. Nyernila Koories Kila Degaia: listen up to Koories speak about health. Koori Heritage Trust Incorporated and Onemda*. VicHealth Koori Health Unit.

Wain, T., Sim., M., Bessarab, D., Mak, D., Hayward, C & Rudd, C. (2016). *Engaging Australian Aboriginal Narratives to Challenge Attitudes and Create Empathy in Health Care: A Methodological Perspective*. BMC Medical Education.

Wampold, B. E. (2001). *The Great Psychotherapy Debate: Models, Methods, and Findings*. Lawrence Erlbaum Associates Publishers.

White, M. & Epston, D. (1990). *Narrative Means to Therapeutic Ends*. New York: W.W. Norton.

World Health Organization. (2020). *Social Determinants of Health*. Geneva: World Health Organization. Retrieved from www.who.int/teams/social-determinants-of-health.

13 Bringing Whānau Ora to Health Social Work

Amohia Boulton, Lynley Cvitanovic and Tracey Cropp

Introduction

This chapter explains the rationale for a Māori-driven social work approach in New Zealand (NZ). It describes the historical, social and political context and challenges for Māori, demonstrating why there is a need for vigilant advocacy and collaboration. The negative health experiences of Māori parallel those experienced by other Indigenous peoples who have been subject to colonisation. A NZ health social work approach offers a unique practice model that may have relevance for other countries.

Why Whānau Ora?

The detrimental impacts of colonisation on Māori, the Indigenous population of NZ, have been well documented. Health impacts include shorter life spans when compared to the overall population (Department of the Prime Minister and Cabinet 2021; Waitangi Tribunal 2019) along with differential access to health care services (Cram 2014), and in the types of treatment offered when Māori present to services for care (Gurney, et al. 2020). Poorer education, justice, employment, and housing outcomes are also apparent (Boulton, et al. 2020; Te Puni Kōkiri 2016a).

Within this broader context of colonisation, social work – along with other caring professions – has often failed to address the needs of Māori. Moyle (2013), for example, describes a dearth of Māori practitioners, and of culturally relevant social work practice, in the field of statutory child protection contributing to detrimental outcomes for whanau.[1] Whereas only a quarter of NZ children identify as Māori, over 65% of those in state care are Māori (Children's Commissioner 2020). The Children's Commissioner (2020:15) unequivocally states 'evidence shows the statutory care and protection system is not working for Māori, and repeated attempts to improve the system have failed'. Bell (2006) identifies oppressive practice targeting Māori clients across a range of state sector social services.[2]

The public sector is the dominant funder and provider of health and social services as well as the leading employer of registered social workers, and of other caring professionals. Almost half of the registered social work workforce is employed by state agencies that include Oranga Tamariki Ministry for Children[3] and District Health Boards (DHBs).[4]

Whānau Ora, broadly translated as the wellbeing of the extended family, is a public policy approach launched in 2010 aimed at improving the responsiveness of the wider social services to Māori (NZ Productivity Commission 2015). The approach recognises that Māori are more than simply the passive recipients of care and must have a far more

DOI: 10.4324/9781003330745-16

active role in shaping service provision. For the purposes of this discussion, Whānau Ora (capitalised) is used to refer specifically to the government's Whānau Ora approach to service delivery, particularly as outlined in the *Whānau Ora Taskforce Report* (2010), and to initiatives arising from this approach such as the funding of specific Whānau Ora providers. However, the term 'whānau ora' (non-capitalised) is used to refer to the philosophy of whānau ora and to any other approach to whānau ora, or a state of wellbeing, more generally.

The constitutional context for government service provision is, in part, established by the Treaty of Waitangi, the founding document of the country, signed by Māori and the Crown in 1840. As our social services are largely funded and delivered by government, the partnership relationship between the Crown and Māori, established by the Treaty, is of particular significance (NZ Productivity Commission 2015). In the years since the signing, breaches of the Treaty have been commonplace. Recent governments have, for a variety of reasons,[5] sought to redress those breaches through the enactment of three treaty principles – partnership, participation and protection – established by the NZ courts, with a view to reducing inequalities and improving wellbeing outcomes for Māori (Boulton et al. 2004, 2013). The NZ Public Health and Disability Act 2000 enshrined the Treaty of Waitangi in social policy legislation for the first time. This landmark legislation sought to increase participation by Māori in the health sector; provided mechanisms to enable Māori to contribute to decision-making about, and delivery of, health and disability services; and charged DHBs with taking responsibility for improving Māori health (Boulton et al. 2004).

Despite these legislative aspirations there have been limited improvements in Māori health, with the system's ability to deliver equity for Māori remaining problematic. A review commissioned by government in 2018 sought to determine the changes necessary to achieve equity and Pae Ora[6] across the system (Department of the Prime Minister and Cabinet 2021). The review's recommendations called for a 'seismic shift' to ensure that the system accurately reflects the principles of the Treaty (Health and Disability System Review 2020).

Reforms announced by government in 2021, in response to the recommendations, are inevitably coloured by both the global and the national COVID-19 pandemic experiences. Jensen et al. (2021:1) describe 'the radically uneven distribution of the health, social and economic risks associated with the pandemic – and the public health measures implemented in response—both within and between societies ... the deep inequities laid bare'.

Successful Māori-led initiatives to protect Māori communities, independently spearheaded by Māori from the earliest days of the pandemic, underline that Māori leadership can drive the achievement of health equity. Building on, and learning from, these successes is a key driver for the positive change signalled in the recently announced public health system reforms (Department of the Prime Minister and Cabinet 2021). The reforms aim to facilitate equity of access and outcomes for Māori, 'simplify' the system, ensure that Iwi[7] and Māori have significantly more control over how services are designed and delivered and give 'real effect to Te Tiriti' (Department of the Prime Minister and Cabinet 2021:7). Indeed, effecting an authentic partnership model for health, whereby the conditions are established under which Māori can exercise self-determination and autonomy through the control of the legislative, regulatory, policy and funding context in which health care is provided is arguably the only means by which equity of health outcome will be achieved (Boulton 2021).

Whānau Ora: Concept and Policy

The concept of whānau ora is complex and based on traditional Māori ways of understanding wellbeing (Kara et al. 2011). It therefore long preceded the 2010 launch of the government's Whānau Ora public policy approach. In simple terms, the concept recognises that the wellbeing of the whole shapes the wellbeing of its constituent parts with whānau having inherent strengths and aspirations to be nurtured (Bpac NZ 2011). Whānau ora is locally defined rather than universally defined and therefore 'may have as many different interpretations as there are Māori tribes and sub-tribes' (Boulton et al. 2013:28).

In the public health and welfare policy domain, the concept of whānau ora was first introduced earlier this century as the core principle of Māori health policy. Boulton et al. (2004) observe that in positioning whānau ora at the centre of its national Māori health strategy, *He Korowai Oranga*, in 2001, the government for the very first time sought to address all elements of Māori health in a single strategy. However, no clear operational definition of whānau ora was contained in *He Korowai Oranga* contributing to implementation challenges (Boulton et al. 2004).

Supported by the advent of DHBs, and their capacity to purchase external services to meet the needs of their communities, the numbers of Kaupapa Māori[8] primary health care (PHC) services grew exponentially from a total of just 20 in 1993 (Boulton et al. 2004). During the 1990s too, with a government focus on devolution of social service provision, iwi entities along with pan-tribal organisations were increasingly positioned to gain contracts for services once provided primarily by state agencies (Rickard 2014). Many of these organisations offer services in their communities and have, since their inception, worked in whānau ora ways as defined by their communities (Moyle 2013). While noting the innovative nature of government's Whānau Ora policy, Rickard (2014) observes the significant influence that practice has had on policy development with Whānau Ora simply 'catching up to the reality of Māori social services provision' (Rickard 2014:48).

Since the introduction of whānau ora into the mainstream[9] public space as the goal for Māori health, the concept has been further developed in the social service services arena most recently with the launch of the Whānau Ora public policy approach (Boulton et al. 2013). In tracing the emergence of Whānau Ora, the NZ Productivity Commission (2015) draws attention to the influence of Māori development initiatives in the social services sector and to *Pūao-te-Āta-tū*, the report of the Ministerial Advisory Committee on a Māori Perspective for the Department of Social Welfare (1986).[10] That report delivered a scathing review of Pākehā[11] and mainstream social work racism detailing 'racist assimilation policies which denied Māori freedoms promised under the Treaty of Waitangi and imposed a welfare dependency status on a people crushed by economic defeat' (McDonald 1998:15).

The advisory committee travelled the country hearing submissions on many marae,[12] as well as in other venues, in order to inform its subsequent recommendations to government. It later recounted the overwhelmingly negative feedback about the department, and its way of working with Māori, repeatedly voiced during the submissions process (Garlick 2012). Rickard (2014) observes that the institutional racism identified in the department's way of working was considered to be reflective of racism across the wider community including other government agencies. *Pūao-te-Āta-tū* was accepted in full by the minister and implementation of the report's recommendations began soon after. By 1996 however, implementation had ground to a halt.

Despite the stalling of the implementation of *Pūao-te-Āta-tū's* recommendations, the mana[13] of those who led the committee's review and the 'extensive hui[14] process' (NZ Productivity Commission 2015:6) involved has contributed to its lasting impact. That impact includes the influence on twenty-first-century views around Māori management and delivery of social services for Māori and is reflected in the prompting of emergent Indigenous social work models of practice 'based on principles of bicultural justice and dignity' (McDonald 1998:15). Indeed Hollis-English (2012a:41) describes *Pūao-te-Āta-tū* as 'the founding document of Māori social work[15] in NZ, second only to Te Tiriti o Waitangi'.

The NZ Productivity Commission (2015) notes repeated references to *Pūao-te-Āta-tū*, throughout its own submission process, as the source of answers as to how best to frame and deliver services that better meet Māori needs. Boulton et al. (2020) too highlight repeated references to the relevance of *Pūao-te-Āta-tū* in major reviews, over the past three decades, focused on issues of critical importance for Māori. *Pūao-te-Āta-tū* identifies that devolution of responsibility for Māori wellbeing to Māori is pivotal to effective services. Devolution, of service delivery whereby iwi/Māori exercise greater autonomy over service design and implementation is an aspirational goal of any Whānau Ora approach. Indeed, with the advent of the COVID-19 pandemic now more than ever *Pūao-te-Āta-tū* provides the blueprint for how we can achieve social equity (Boulton et al. 2020).

The Government's Whānau Ora Approach

In 2010, the Taskforce on Whānau Centred Initiatives (TWCI) released its report calling for the reconfiguration of the public sector and not for profit (NFP) agencies working with whānau along with the use of a whānau ora approach by these agencies (Kara et al. 2011). The taskforce identified an overarching Whānau Ora framework described by Boulton et al. (2013:25) as 'being at once a philosophy, a model of practice and an outcome'. Derived both from Māori values and beliefs and from public policy best practice, seven principles comprise the framework. These principles are cognisant of the Treaty of Waitangi, acknowledging that both Māori and the Crown share in the responsibility for achieving whānau wellbeing or whānau ora, and are:

- ngā kaupapa tuku iho (Māori values, beliefs, obligations and responsibilities guide whānau in their day-to-day lives);
- whānau opportunity (to be part of their communities and socially connected);
- best whānau outcomes (whānau empowered to live healthy lives and achieve optimum wellbeing);
- whānau integrity (recognition and acceptance of whānau accountability, dignity and ability to facilitate their own transformation);
- coherent service delivery (integrated service provision in the best interests of whānau);
- effective resourcing (scoped to the work to be carried out with whānau and clearly linked to achieving outcomes); and
- competent and innovative provision (recognising the need for skilled and creative practitioners committed to whānau empowerment and to supporting whānau transformation) (Boulton et al. 2013).

The principles underpin broader outcome goals which identify that whānau will be:

- self-managing;
- living healthy lifestyles;
- participating fully in society;
- participating confidently in Te Ao Māori[16] communities;
- economically secure and successfully involved in wealth creation; and
- cohesive, resilient and nurturing (Taskforce on Whānau Centred Initiatives 2010).

A seventh outcome, that whānau will be responsible stewards of their living and natural environments, was added in 2015 by the Whānau Ora Partnership Group. This joint Crown-Iwi governance body was established in 2014 to provide Whānau Ora strategic governance. The Group included both Te Tiriti partners, that is, six iwi leaders and six Crown Ministers (Te Puni Kōkiri 2016b) reflecting a commitment on the part of both parties to better integrate services to support a whānau service delivery focus (NZ Government 2014).

A 2018 government commissioned review endorsed and reaffirmed Whānau Ora, recommending its continued growth. The review identified the pivotal role of the partnership group in ensuring Māori-Crown partnership in the oversight of Whānau Ora (Office of the Minister for Whānau Oraa 2019).

Implementing the Government's Whānau Ora Policy Approach

In brief, Whānau Ora has been rolled out in two overlapping phases. During phase one (2010–2014) funding streams were established and administered through government agency Te Puni Kōkiri (TPK), the Ministry of Māori Development. One stream aimed to strengthen the Whānau Ora capability of Māori health and social services providers. Another allowed contracted providers to appoint Whānau Ora practitioners, or kaiārahi, to work alongside whānau to plan for achieving or maintaining wellbeing and to support implementing whānau plans.

In phase two (2014 to present) responsibility for achieving Whānau Ora outcomes was devolved from TPK to three NFP commissioning agencies. These agencies were established and contracted by TPK for an initial period of three years (1 July 2014 to 30 June 2017) (NZ Productivity Commission 2015). All have continued to hold Whānau Ora contracts with TPK subsequent to the initial funding period.

Replacement of the National Coalition government by a Labour-led government, late in 2017, saw a significant shift in the Whānau Ora model with the formal dissolution of the Whānau Ora Partnership Group. That dissolution seriously undermined the previous government's commitment to better integrate services to support a whānau service delivery focus (Boulton 2019); removed the strategic leadership that had, to date driven the implementation of the policy; and effectively reduced the focus of the policy solely to service provision, rather than a whole of government approach aimed at improving wellbeing outcomes for Māori.

What Is Distinctive about the Whānau Ora Policy Approach?

Being underpinned by Māori values, and a Māori worldview of wellbeing, Whānau Ora is unique to NZ. It is an innovative initiative that arguably signals the strongest public policy move to date to shift social services commissioning and delivery for Māori away from a mainstream approach, ostensibly designed to serve the entire population but primarily reflective of Pākehā interests, to a 'by Māori approach for Māori' approach; an approach that facilitates culturally meaningful service provision.

Although Whānau Ora stops short of allocating resources directly to Māori control, it nevertheless represents a significant shift in the public policy space. That shift validates the work Māori providers do to support holistic, whānau centred care despite the constraints of operating in a wider funding and contracting environment more conducive to supporting care through services to individuals and in silos (Boulton et al. 2013).

Our approach to social services delivery is characterised by tightly prescribed provision through a range of separate and largely uncoordinated government agencies and government funded providers primarily in the NFP sector (NZ Productivity Commission 2015). A key aim of Whānau Ora is to broker ways of negotiating service fragmentation at a range of levels, including at whānau level; internally at local provider and agency level; at local interagency and inter-provider level; and at central government level. At whānau level, negotiation may occur through working alongside whānau to navigate the complexities of government agency and NFP sector provision to access the services that work best for whānau as determined by whānau themselves. At both the local and central government levels, Whānau Ora advocates for the integration of service provision.

Whānau Ora in Practice

How Whānau Ora 'works' in practice is conditioned by a multitude of factors including whānau preference and a particular provider's approach. Whānau may elect to make use of a provider's Whānau Ora kaiārahi. A Māori service provider manager highlights the uniqueness of kaiārahi:

> The difference between a ... [kaiārahi] who can go into the home, speak the language of the whānau, engage in a way that's meaningful and still leave them with their mana intact [and a worker who is not able to do these things] cannot be underestimated ... We have people who are used to being in a health setting or a social work setting which are really valuable skills but sometimes they don't access whānau in a way that leaves the whānau with a mana enhancing experience.
>
> (Grant 2015)

Kaiārahi support whānau to identify their own priorities and strengths and to plan for achieving their desired outcomes. Whānau may, with the input of the kaiārahi, bring together the services and other support they decide is needed to reach their goals. The services used are likely to range widely and may, for example, include housing and employment services (Te Puni Kōkiri 2016a) that would ordinarily need to be separately accessed requiring whānau to repeatedly recount their stories in each instance. Other whānau may choose to develop their own plans for enhanced whānau outcomes and to work on those plans with the support of hapū,[17] iwi or a Māori organisation other than a services provider.

To further illustrate the nature of whānau ora intervention, two case study examples are explored below.[18] The first concerns Whānau Ora activity under the umbrella of Te Oranganui Trust,[19] a Māori governed and led Whānau Ora-funded provider operating in the Whanganui DHB region of NZ.[20] The second explores whānau ora work carried out under the umbrella of Hospice, a mainstream NFP organisation in the same region.

Reflection: Rawiri's Story

Rawiri was living 'rough' in a derelict building after his kuia[21] who had raised him, in another part of the country, died. Struggling to deal with his grief, Rawiri had shut people out and chosen to leave town. Now he found himself broke and far from home. He was hungry and socially isolated, with no whānau around him. The police charged Rawiri with unlawfully being on private property. He was handed a community-based sentence requiring him to work at a local marae on specified days. At the marae, he met the local Whānau Ora provider's kaiārahi.

With strong links in the local community through her iwi and hapū affiliations, the kaiārahi often visited the marae where Rawiri worked. She sensed he was struggling emotionally and spiritually. She eventually learned of his living situation and recognised that he was facing critical challenges across all four interconnecting dimensions of his wellbeing: te taha tinana (physical), taha wairua (spiritual), taha hinengaro (mental) and taha whānau (environment/context) (Kara et al. 2011).

Drawing on her connections and cultural knowledge, the kaiārahi slowly eased Rawiri into the fold of the marae, the hapū and the iwi, using the korowai[22] of the people to wrap around him to create a safe space. The people demonstrated kinship with him by upholding kaitiakitanga[23] and ensuring that he had his immediate basic needs met. Recognising the need too for Rawiri to move through his grieving process, the kaiārahi and the local people supported his spiritual reconnection with his tupuna[24] allowing him to safely send his kuia to the realm of the departed. The kaiārahi supported Rawiri to renew connections with his whānau back home as he worked to restore stability in his life. To address the needs in the physical dimension of his wellbeing longer-term, the kaiārahi linked Rawiri with mainstream community agencies that could support him to establish and maintain a home and an income.

The key features of Rawiri's case are highlighted in Figure 13.1.

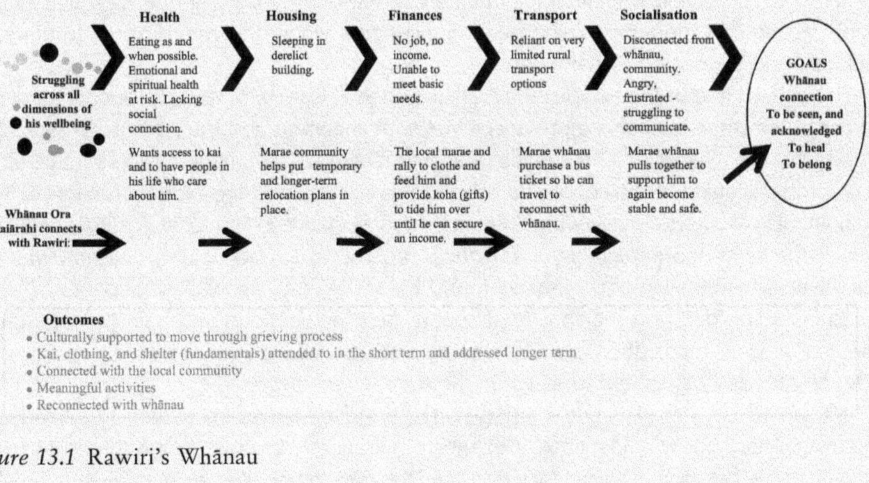

Figure 13.1 Rawiri's Whānau

Reflection: Hinemoa's Story

Hinemoa a 52-year-old mother, grandmother and wife, was diagnosed with cancer six months before presenting at Hospice. She was the full-time caregiver of her 18-month-old granddaughter. She also supported her adult son (the child's father) who was living with her. He was struggling with alcohol and other drug issues and was unable to adequately care for his daughter. The child's mother had died six days after giving birth. Oranga Tamariki placed the child in Hinemoa's care after removing her from her maternal whānau following safety concerns.

Hinemoa returned to her hometown to be with extended whānau following her diagnosis. She went into the Hospice inpatient unit, for symptom management, when her health began to rapidly decline. Hinemoa was faced with multiple challenges during her initial two week stay. These challenges included the breakdown of her marriage when her husband (not the paternal grandparent) returned her grandchild to the maternal whānau without her authority. The unauthorised handover necessitated Oranga Tamariki intervention. Hinemoa's son was also admitted to alcohol and other drug inpatient services during this time and the findings of the coroner's inquest into the death of her daughter-in-law were due to be announced. Additionally, she needed enduring power of attorney in place should she be unable to make decisions regarding her welfare and property.

Due to Hinemoa's rapid decline, it was evident that she would need a trusted spokesperson to represent her interests. A whānau hui was convened during which Hinemoa asked a cousin to be her spokesperson and advocate. The Hospice kaiārahi co-ordinated the whānau hui that included other Hospice staff. Hinemoa's whānau led the hui beginning with a ruruku[25] to bring comfort, to acknowledge those in the spiritual realm who have come before, those present and those who will follow. The ruruku helped to alleviate fear and anxiety, to bring strength and clarity to the end-of-life journey and to ensure a smooth hui process.

The medical officer shared clinical information with whānau, with Hinemoa's permission. In this safe setting, she talked about her immediate needs and the things impacting on her emotional wellbeing including the care of her grandchild, her marriage issues, her son's issues and the support she needed. Hinemoa wanted to return home to die surrounded and supported by her whānau.

The agreed role of the Hospice kaiārahi included liaising with the appropriate services to assist Hinemoa; all service providers met with Hinemoa and the kaiārahi at Hospice. They included a Whānau Ora service, a lawyer, Oranga Tamariki and representatives of the coroner's office, the alcohol and other drugs service and the probation service. The kaiārahi also worked closely with Hinemoa, her whānau and the local Whānau Ora service to develop and implement a whānau wraparound support plan. Hinemoa was no longer able to mobilise and required round the clock support with all aspects of daily living including decision making, full support with medications and pain management. Medical aids, a medication plan, a nursing and medical officer roster, an ambulance plan and funded caregivers to assist in the home were arranged.

Within two days of Hinemoa's return home, the need for an immediate Hospice team interdisciplinary hui was identified. Hinemoa's estranged daughter had returned to town wanting to be her mother's primary caregiver. However, other whānau were already providing care including several kuia. Hinemoa's daughter was unwilling to take guidance from her

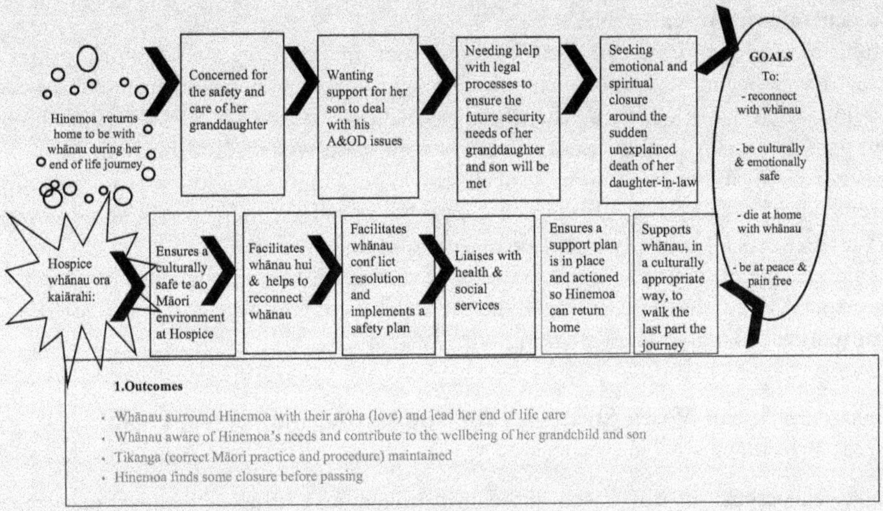

Figure 13.2 Hinemoa's Whānau

kuia, and appeared unable to readily identify her mother's needs, creating significant conflict in the home.

The Hospice kaiārahi facilitated a hui at Hinemoa's home with the whānau to find some resolution but this was unsuccessful. Hinemoa's spokesperson was therefore immediately contacted. Following discussion with her, the spokesperson arranged with the kaiārahi for Hinemoa to immediately return to the Hospice inpatient unit. Back at Hospice, the kaiārahi worked closely with Hinemoa and her whānau to ensure they were wrapped within the korowai; this is symbolic of leadership and includes the obligation to care for people and environment taking account of emotional, spiritual, physical and whānau wellbeing.

Hinemoa passed away soon after her return to Hospice; at peace, pain-free and surrounded by her whānau. Time and facilities were made available so the whānau could stay with Hinemoa following her passing. Her spokesperson provided guidance on the tangi[26] preparations while Hospice collated the necessary documentation and contacted the funeral director the whānau had chosen.

Water was placed outside Hinemoa's room so that the whānau was able to practice whakawaatea 'the sprinkling of water on self to leave the spirit to follow their own journey home'. Candles were lit in the inpatient unit and also in the reception area, to alert others that someone in residence had died. The Hospice staff created a protective space to surround Hinemoa and her whānau as they left.

After Hinemoa left, the kaiārahi opened the windows and doors of her now empty room and blessed the space with karakia to support the essence or mauri[27] to continue on their journey. The room was then left for 24 hours to rest.

Whānau Ora and Mainstream Social Work

In reflecting on both the local level provider philosophy of whānau ora, and on kaiārahi practice under the umbrella of whānau ora-contracted providers, we suggest that the key principles of whānau ora contrast markedly with those underpinning mainstream social work generally in Aotearoa NZ.

Munford and Sanders (2011:74) contend that mainstream social work policy and practice have 'begun to explore the ways in which they can incorporate Māori worldviews into their work'. Indeed, the findings of Puao-Te-Ata-Tu (1988), which highlight the impact of racism in this country both within state welfare and beyond, have been a significant catalyst for beginning a social work paradigm shift away from a dominant Western model (Boulton & Cvitanovic 2021). Nevertheless, there is still some way to go if mainstream social work is to better meet the needs of whānau.

Table 13.1 identifies some notable areas of difference between whānau ora and mainstream social work that in turn highlight the tensions kaiārahi, Māori social workers and health workers manage when working with whānau.

Mainstream Social Work Strategies for Supporting Indigenous Health and Social Services Providers

Social work practice in NZ is conducted in a unique and complex context; one enmeshed within a dynamic and vital Indigenous culture. Having recognised that the practice of social work here is unique, and that the setting in which it is conducted is complex, it is useful to consider the ways in which mainstream social work may best support service delivery that is responsive to Māori. A role for mainstream social work is particularly critical in light of the reality that the majority of social work-related roles are concentrated in mainstream services and that public sector organisations remain the major service providers (Walsh-Tapiata 2004).

How then can mainstream social work be more responsive to the needs of Māori? As a start we suggest a flexible set of strategies drawing particularly on the work of Walsh-Tapiata (2004) and Ruwhiu (2009). In implementing these strategies in their own practice, mainstream practitioners may achieve the dual aims of enhancing cultural responsiveness within their own agencies along with supporting and upholding the work of Indigenous social service providers. These strategies include:

- Taking responsibility for ongoing learning about our national and regional colonial history from the perspective of the Indigenous population. In Aotearoa NZ learning about the significance of the Treaty of Waitangi, and its historical and contemporary impact, is particularly critical (Ruwhiu 2009, Walsh-Tapiata 2004).
- Respecting the part that narrative, or story-telling plays for Māori, and other Indigenous communities, as a way of putting history and the past into context and 'as a means of explaining their situation' (Walsh-Tapiata 2004:3). Narratives are important in the construction and maintenance of cultural identity as well as being integral to a process of healing (Ruwhiu 2009).
- Being aware of mono-cultural norms shaping practice within (Moyle 2014) and beyond agencies and seeking to name and address these being cognisant of roles in maintaining the status quo as well as of the opportunities available to act as agents of change (Walsh-Tapiata 2004).
- Recognising that the beliefs, values and practices of Indigenous peoples are likely to be different from Western worldviews and practices but are equally valid.
- Recognising that Indigenous colleagues, both within (Moyle 2014) and external to social work agencies, are not responsible for the learning of non-Indigenous practitioners (in relation to, for example, Indigenous worldviews and practices).

Table 13.1 Comparing Whānau ora and mainstream social work in New Zealand

Whānau ora	*Mainstream social work*
Indigenous in its focus (specific to Aotearoa NZ) and in its application. Particular to local contexts as determined by local iwi.	Globally defined practice-based profession and academic discipline with a holistic and universal focus. Amenable to national and regional contexts (International Federation of Social Workers 2014).
Rooted in Māori values and cultural traditions; inherent within Te Ao Māori.	Rooted in British and American social work traditions (McDonald 1998).
Built primarily around traditional Māori cultural knowledge, wisdom and experience drawing on Western theories, models and approaches informing mainstream social work practice where deemed relevant (Hollis 2006; Ruwhiu 2009).	Historically built almost exclusively around Western knowledge – theories, models and approaches.
Cognisant of the Treaty of Waitangi acknowledging that both Māori and the Crown share in the responsibility for achieving whānau wellbeing (Boulton & Cvitanovic 2021).	Increasingly cognisant of the Treaty of Waitangi and implications for practice.
Greater emphasis on collectivism. (Rickard 2014) The wellbeing of the individual is reliant on the collective wellbeing of whānau (Te Moananui-Makirere et al. 2014).	Greater emphasis on individualism.
Whānau-centred; whānau, hapū and iwi pivotal to Māori models of wellbeing (Kara et al. 2011). The wellbeing of the individual is reliant on the collective wellbeing of whānau (Te Moananui-Makirere et al. 2014).	Draws on family-centred approaches (predominantly on Western concepts of family) and on other approaches including individual and group approaches.
Values and gives priority to a Māori world view when working with Māori (Bell 2006).	Values and is more likely to give priority, consciously or unconsciously, to a dominant Western world view when working with Māori.
Whānau safety, including cultural, physical, emotional and spiritual safety, is a priority (Kara et al. 2011).	Client safety is a priority.
Focused on interrelated dimensions of wellbeing as understood by Māori. Draws on Māori models that highlight the interplay of spirituality, language, ancestral land and community (Kara et al. 2011).	May focus on one or more dimensions of wellbeing (commonly drawing exclusively on Western understandings of what constitutes wellbeing).
Collective self-determination/whānau self-determination. Seeks to position whānau as self-sufficient networks providing for their own social support needs interdependently and on their own terms (Bell 2006; Savage et al. 2017; Walsh-Tapiata 2004).	Client self-determination. Empowers clients to independently access and utilise services and networks to address their social support needs.
Whānau concept of confidentiality takes priority.	Western individual concept of confidentiality takes priority.
Practice influenced by a Māori cultural milieu (organisation and setting).	Practice influenced by the dominant Pākehā cultural milieu.
Embedded in iwi and Māori organisations, agencies and groups.	Concentrated primarily in public sector health and social services and in the mainstream NFP sector.

Whānau ora	*Mainstream social work*
Emphasises that every whānau has strengths, along with aspirations and the potential to achieve them.	May draw on a strengths-based approach.
Growing connections within and across whānau supporting wellbeing through interdependence.	Supporting social connectedness to enhance wellbeing.
Integrated, cross-sector focus.	Settings-based/distinct fields of practice (e.g. family harm, refugee resettlement, aged care).
Assumes that practitioners who identify as Māori are best positioned to successfully connect with whānau and contribute to enhancing whānau wellbeing.	Assumes that appropriately trained, credentialled and professionally supervised practitioners can work effectively across client groups.
Enhances and/or restores the mana of the whānau through the process of realising the moemoea (dreams and aspirations) of the whānau (Savage et al. 2017).	Respect central to working relationships with individuals, groups, families and communities.
Cultural understanding and relational skills a priority (Rickard 2014). Draws practitioners from across health and social services professions as well as from kaimahi[28] groupings such as community health workers.	Regulated, professionalised and qualifications based.
Building Māori provider and whānau ora capacity to enhance whānau interdependence and wellbeing; including developing a critical analysis of colonisation and facilitating a process of decolonisation (Bell 2006).	Building and maintaining professional competencies to enhance client wellbeing.
Local (whānau) connections and iwi knowledge pivotal.	Local connections (networks) and local knowledge relevant.

- Building and continuing to develop understanding of concepts critical to Indigenous peoples (Ruwhiu 2009).
- Building and sustaining mana-enhancing relationships with local Whānau Ora providers and other Indigenous providers with a view to opening doors to services and resources for the benefit of whanau.
- Being open to observe, to listen and to learn (Hyslop 2016).

Conclusion

While mainstream social work skills and knowledge are likely to be of use to the Whānau Ora practitioner, it is apparent that social work alone is not enough to support competent practice in the whānau ora space. Cram (2012) draws attention to international research that seeks to understand the complexities which give rise to the significant overrepresentation of Indigenous children in care globally. She highlights the pivotal role of institutional, or systemic, racism which privileges a white, middle-class view of what family means and how family life should be conducted. Indigenous values and practices measured against these dominant norms are commonly found wanting. The 'intergenerational fragmentation of the family and community structure resulting from past assimilation-oriented government policies with respect to [indigenous] child welfare' (Cram 2012:11) exacerbates an already fraught situation for Indigenous communities striving to retain their children in their care.

In 2015 the government announced its intent to restructure its CYF service in order to better address state care of Māori children. The minister for social development established a Modernising Child Youth and Family Expert Panel and charged it with developing a new child-centric operating model for CYF (Ministry of Social Development 2015). The panel later recommended that a Ministry for Vulnerable Children be established to replace CYF (Ministry of Social Development 2016). Vocal opposition from Māori and non-Māori leaders, academics, researchers, community and social workers resulted. That opposition centred around the labelling of a ministry predicated upon deficit approaches to child welfare and with scant regard for cultural context (Te Wharepora Hou: Māori Women's Network 2016). Despite the scale of opposition, the new ministry became operational early in 2017. By the close of that year however, a Labour government assumed power and swiftly oversaw the deletion of the term 'vulnerable' from the name of the new ministry.

Despite renaming the child care and protection agency *Oranga Tamariki*, meaning 'child wellbeing', we suggest that the likelihood of turning around the significantly disparate levels of tamariki Māori in state care is minimal without the embedment of Whānau Ora as the primary way of working with whānau. Indeed, early indications are that, despite an organisational name change reflecting, at least on the surface, a better understanding of whānau dynamics and needs, mana-enhancing social work practice within the organisation has yet to become the norm. In conclusion, Whānau Ora, given the necessary space and opportunity by the state and the NFP sector, offers an alternative pathway for Māori whānau; one which affirms the Treaty of Waitangi (Cram 2012) and offers support, hope and solutions on Māori terms drawing on the strengths inherent within a Māori way of being.

Key Website Resources

Office of the Children's Commissioner (www.occ.org.nz).
Te Pou Matakana (www.tepoumatakana.com).
Te Puni Kōkiri (www.tpk.govt.nz).
Te Wharepora Hou: Māori Women's Network (https://tewhareporahou.wordpress.com).

Notes

1 Whānau: a horizontally and vertically extended family grouping connected by descent from a common ancestor.
2 Bell (2006) contends, for example, that statutory social work is commonly viewed by Māori as another tool of colonisation creating whānau dependency on the state, isolating children from their whānau and cultural heritage and failing to effectively engage whānau in decision making about the wellbeing of dependants.
3 Government agency responsible for ensuring that children and youth are safe and nurtured in their families, whānau and homes.
4 DHBs provide and fund hospital and other health services at the regional level (Careers NZ 2021).
5 Including in response to the Māori cultural renaissance which began in the 1970s (Moyle 2013; Rickard 2014).
6 Pae Ora is a holistic concept encompassing the three inextricably linked elements of healthy individuals (mauri ora), healthy families (whānau ora) and healthy environments (wai ora).
7 Iwi: extended kinship group or tribe.
8 Kaupapa Māori services carry out their work with whānau 'based on Māori cultural values, processes and beliefs' (Boulton et al. 2013:22).

9 The term 'mainstream' is used here to refer to the underpinning worldview, values, systems, and processes of the culturally and numerically dominant population of NZ; the population made up of those of Western European descent.
10 The Department of Social Welfare was dismantled in the late 1990s when several stand-alone agencies were created including the Children, Young Persons and their Families Agency (Garlick 2012), since renamed Oranga Tamariki Ministry for Children.
11 Pākehā: NZer of European descent.
12 Marae: traditional meeting place for whānau, hapū and/ or iwi.
13 Mana: respect, authority, status, integrity.
14 Hui: meeting.
15 Hollis-English (2012b:17) notes that Māori social work includes 'knowledge that has come out of Te Ao Māori, the various contemporary methods and models that have been developed, and the ability to adapt these to the various Māori families within Aotearoa NZ'. Māori models of practice are identified and discussed by many others including, for example, Bell (2006), Eruera (2012), King (2014) and Te Moananui-Makirere et al. (2014).
16 Te Ao Māori: Māori worldview.
17 Hapū: subtribe.
18 Anonymised and partially aggregated for the purposes of this discussion.
19 Te Oranganui provides services that include primary health care, whānau and community support and disability support (Te Oranganui 2021).
20 The WDHB region covers a population of approximately 68,400 people, a higher population of Māori (27.3 per cent) than the national average (16.6 per cent) and proportionally significantly more people in the most deprived section of the population (Ministry of Health 2021).
21 Kuia: grandmother, female elder.
22 Korowai: cloak. The term is used metaphorically here to denote concepts of care and protection.
23 Kaitiakitanga: responsible trusteeship.
24 Tupuna: ancestors, forebears.
25 Ruruku: blessing.
26 Tangi: Māori funeral rite.
27 Mauri: spirit.
28 Kaimahi: worker.

References

Bell, H. (2006). Exiting the matrix: colonisation, decolonisation and social work in Aotearoa. Voices of Ngāti Raukawa Ki Te Tonga Kaimahi Whānau. Master of philosophy thesis, Massey University. Retrieved from https://mro.massey.ac.nz/bitstream/handle/10179/662/02whole.pdf?sequence=1&isAllowed=y.

Boulton, A. (2019). Whānau Ora: A culturally-informed, social policy innovation. *NZ Sociology* 34(2), 23–48.

Boulton, A. (2021). Māori governance in the NZ health system. In R. Joseph & R. Benton (eds), *Waking the Taniwha: Māori governance in the twenty-first century* (pp. 449–469). Thompson Reuters.

Boulton, A. & Cvitanovic, L. (2021). *Māori centred social work practice: Evidence brief.* Wellington, NZ: Oranga Tamariki Evidence Centre, Oranga Tamariki Ministry for Children.

Boulton, A., Levy, M., Cvitanovic, L. (2020). Beyond puao te ata tū: realising the promise of a new day. Retrieved from www.maramatanga.ac.nz/sites/default/files/teArotahi_20-1106.pdf.

Boulton, A., Simonsen, K., Walker, T., Cumming, J. & Cunningham, C. (2004). Indigenous participation in the 'new' NZ health structure. *Journal of Health Services Research and Policy*, 9 (Supplement 2), 35–40.

Boulton, A., Tamehana, J. and Brannelly, P. M. (2013). Whānau-centred health and social service delivery in NZ: the challenges to, and opportunities for, innovation. *MAI Journal: A NZ Journal of Indigenous Scholarship*, 2(1), 18–32.

Bpac NZ. (2011). Whānau Ora: the theory and the practice. *Best Practice Journal*, 37. Retrieved from www.bpac.org.nz/BPJ/2011/august/whanau_ora.aspx.

Careers NZ. (2021). Jobs database. Retrieved from www.careers.govt.nz/jobs-database/health-and-community/community-services/social-worker.

Children's Commissioner. (2020). *Briefing to the incoming minister*. Wellington, Aotearoa NZ: Office of the Children's Commissioner.

Cram, F. (2012). *Safety of subsequent children – Māori children and whānau: a review of selected literature*. Wellington, Aotearoa NZ: Families Commission Kōmihana ā Whānau.

Cram, F. (2014). *Improving Māori access to health care: Research Report*. Wellington: Ministry of Health.

Department of the Prime Minister and Cabinet. (2021). Our health and disability system: Building a stronger health and disability system that delivers for all NZers. Retrieved from https://dpmc.govt.nz/sites/default/files/2021-04/heallth-reform-white-paper-summary-apr21.pdf.

Eruera, M. (2012). He kōrari, he kete, he kōrero. *Te Komako*, 24(3–4), 12–19. Retrieved from https://anzswjournal.nz/anzsw/article/view/103.

Garlick, T. (2012). *Social developments: an organisational history of the Ministry of Social Development and its predecessors, 1860–2011*. Wellington, Aotearoa NZ: Steele Roberts Aotearoa. Retrieved from www.msd.govt.nz/documents/about-msd-and-our-work/about-msd/history/social-developments.pdf.

Grant, N. (2015). *How important are kaiārahi to whānau success?*Auckland, Aotearoa NZ: Te Pou Matakana.

Gurney, J., Stanley, J., McLeod, M., Koea, J., Jackson, C. & Sarfati, D. (2020). Disparities in cancer-specific survival between Māori and non-Māori NZers, 2007–2016. *JCO Global Oncology*, 6, 766–774.

Health and Disability System Review. (2020). *Health and Disability System Review – Final Report – Pūrongo Whakamutunga*. Wellington: HDSR.

Hollis, A. (2006). Pūao-te-Āta-tū and Māori social work methods. Master's thesis, University of Otago. Retrieved from https://ourarchive.otago.ac.nz/bitstream/handle/10523/175/HollisAwhina2005MA.pdf?sequence=4&isAllowed=y.

Hollis-English, A. (2012a). Pūao-te-Āta-tū: informing Māori social work since 1986. *Aotearoa NZ Social Work*, 24(3–4), 41–48.

Hollis-English, A. (2012b). Māori social workers: experiences within social service organisations. Doctoral dissertation, University of Otago. Retrieved from https://ourarchive.otago.ac.nz/bitstream/handle/10523/2127/HollisEnglishAwhinaNR2012PhD.pdf?sequence=1&isAllowed=y.

Hyslop, I. (2016, 5 January). Racism and social work in Aotearoa NZ: a Pākehā perspective. Retrieved from www.reimaginingsocialwork.nz/2016/01/racism-and-social-work-in-aotearoa-new-zealand-a-pakeha-perspective/.

International Federation of Social Workers. (2014). Global definition of social work. Retrieved from http://ifsw.org/policies/definition-of-social-work.

Jensen, N., Kelly, A. & Avendano, N. (2021). The COVID-19 pandemic underscores the need for an equity-focused global health agenda. *Humanities and Social Sciences Communications*, 8, 15.

Kara, E., Gibbons, V., Kidd, J., Blundell, R., Turner, K. & Johnstone, W. (2011). Developing a kaupapa Māori framework for whānau ora. *AlterNative: An International Journal of Indigenous Peoples*, 7(2), 100–110.

King, L. (2014). KIAORA – the emerging construction of a bicultural professional supervision model. *Te Aotearoa NZ Social Work*, 16(1), 20–28. Retrieved from https://anzswjournal.nz/anzsw/article/view/51.

McDonald, D. (1998). *Social work in Aotearoa NZ: an introduction*. Auckland, Aotearoa NZ: Addison Wesley Longman.

Ministerial Advisory Committee on a Māori Perspective for the Development of Social Welfare. (1988). *Puao-te-Ata-tu*. Wellington NZ: Ministerial Advisory Committee on a Māori Perspective for the Development of Social Welfare.

Ministry of Health. (2021). Population of Whanganui DHB. Retrieved from www.health.govt.nz/new-zealand-health-system/my-dhb/whanganui-dhb/population-whanganui-dhb.

Ministry of Social Development. (2015). *Modernising child, youth and family.* Wellington, Aotearoa NZ: Ministry of Social Development.

Ministry of Social Development. (2016). *New children's agency established – the Ministry for Vulnerable Children, Oranga Tamariki.* Wellington, Aotearoa NZ: Ministry of Social Development.

Moyle, P. (2013). From family group conferencing to Whānau Ora: Māori social workers talk about their experiences. Master's thesis, Massey University. Retrieved from http://mro.massey.ac.nz/bitstream/handle/10179/4731/02_whole.pdf?sequence=1.

Moyle, P. (2014). Māori social workers' experiences of care and protection: a selection of findings. *Te Komako, Social Work Review*, 26(1), 55–64. Retrieved from https://anzswjournal.nz/anzsw/article/view/55.

Munford, R. & Sanders, J. (2011). Embracing the diversity of practice: indigenous knowledge and mainstream social work practice. *Journal of Social Work Practice*, 25(1), 63–77.

NZ Government. (2014). Iwi members appointed to Whānau Ora group. Retrieved from www.beehive.govt.nz/release/iwi-members-appointed-wh%C4%81nau-ora-group.

NZ Productivity Commission. (2015). More effective social services. Retrieved from www.productivity.govt.nz/sites/default/files/social-services-final-report-main.pdf.

Office of the Minister for Whānau Oraa. (2019). *Proactive release of initial response to the review of Whānau Ora.* [Cabinet Paper]. Wellington, Aotearoa NZ: NZ Government.

Rickard, T. (2014). He iwi moke, he whanokē Iwi social services, policy and practice. Unpublished master's thesis, Massey University. Retrieved from http://mro.massey.ac.nz/bitstream/handle/10179/5768/02_whole.pdf?sequence=2&.

Ruwhiu, L. (2009). Indigenous issues in Aotearoa NZ. In M. Connolly & L. Harms (eds), *Social work context and practice* (2nd edition). Melbourne, Australia: Oxford University Press.

Savage, C., Katoa, W., & Proctor, T. (2017). Whānau Ora navigators initial research for Te Pūtahitanga o Te Waipounamu. Retrieved from https://whanauoraresearch.co.nz/wp-content/uploads/2020/11/6.-NavigatorReport.pdf.

Taskforce on Whānau Centred Initiatives. (2010). *Whānau Ora: report of the Taskforce on Whānau Centred Initiatives.* Report produced for Hon. Tariana Turia, minister for the community and voluntary sector. Wellington, Aotearoa NZ: Ministry of Social Development.

Te Moananui-Makirere, J., King, L, Eruera, M., Tukukino, M., & Maoate-Davis, S. (2014). Te Ara Whakapikoranga. *Aotearoa NZ Social Work*, 26(1), 10–19. Retrieved from https://anzswjournal.nz/anzsw/rt/printerFriendly/50/0.

Te Oranganui. (2021). Te Pūrongo-ā- Tau 2020. Retrieved from www.teoranganui.co.nz/publications.

Te Puni Kōkiri. (2016a). Frequently asked questions. Retrieved from www.tpk.govt.nz/en/whakamahia/whanau-ora/frequently-asked-questions.

Te Puni Kōkiri. (2016b). Whānau Ora outcomes framework. Retrieved from www.tpk.govt.nz/docs/tpk-wo-outcomesframework-aug2016.pdf.

Te Wharepora Hou: Māori Women's Network. (2016). Hands off our Tamariki: An open letter to Whānau, Hapū, Iwi, Iwi Leaders Forum, Māori members of parliament, Māori national and iwi organisations. Retrieved from https://tewhareporahou.wordpress.com/2016/10/09/hands-off-our-tamariki-an-open-letter.

Waitangi Tribunal. (2019). *Hauora: Report on stage one of the Health Services and Outcomes Kaupapa Inquiry: Wai 2575.* Waitangi Tribunal.

Walsh-Tapiata, W. (2004). The past the present and the future: The NZ indigenous experience of social work. Retrieved from http://anzasw.nz/wp-content/uploads/Social-Work-Review-16-Summer-04-Article-Walsh-Tapiata.pdf.

Whanganui District Health Board. (2021). Region & population. Retrieved from www.wdhb.org.nz/about-us/our-region-and-population.

14 Social Work in Health

Considerations for Refugee Health

Kim Robinson

Introduction

Every day we turn on the news and hear about refugees and asylum seekers seeking safety and a better life. In Australia the media has focused on the political manoeuvring of parties, and the policy changes and regulations that restrict movement of families and individuals escaping war and displacement. Competing discourses confront communities as they struggle with how to meet the challenges facing new arrivals in the context of international discord, and now the COVID-19 pandemic, and they have caused deep political and social divisions. Settlement and resettlement practices of international significance include Sanctuary Cities, Cities of Welcome and Solidarity Cities. Social workers are well placed to tackle these challenges and promote human rights and social justice to work effectively directly with service users in organisations and in communities. As social work students and practitioners you will work with some of these service users and encounter a range of complex issues.

This chapter explores the social work practices of working with refugees and asylum seekers.[1] This area of work is perceived as contested ground however critical perspectives both critique and inform social work practice, and social workers can actively work in the delivery of services in a variety of settings (Ife 2016; Nipperess & Williams 2019). Critical theory, anti-oppressive practice, human rights and social justice are just some of the key narratives in this field of practice (Fook 2016; Morley, Ablett & Macfarlane 2019). The chapter will briefly highlight the debates in the literature on mental health and well-being, and how these intersect with the 'doing' of health based social work with refugees and asylum seekers. Examples of lived experience will enable you to reflect on some of the challenges working in this field of social work.

Background to Refugee Programmes

The Australian Government has a commitment to providing support to refugees via its Humanitarian Settlement Program (HSP) (Australian Government, 2021) which establishes an annual quota for entry, based on assessments provided by the United Nations High Commission for Refugees (UNHCR). Services are funded by both Federal and State government and consist of housing, health care, torture and trauma services, education, English language classes and access to benefits. There are five main categories of refugee and humanitarian visas: Refugee visa (Subclass 200); In-country special humanitarian programme (Subclass 201); Emergency rescue visa (Subclass 203) and Women at risk visa (Subclass 204) (Australian Government, 2021). Global special humanitarian programme

DOI: 10.4324/9781003330745-17

(Subclass 201) applicants are ineligible for HSP as they access support via the Community Support Program who sponsors them.

The Special Humanitarian Program (SHP) programme is for people outside Australia who have suffered discrimination amounting to human rights violations and have an individual or organisation in Australia to support their application for resettlement (Australian Government, 2021). Refugees who have been approved and processed prior to arrival onshore, enter under these different categories. In contrast, asylum seekers are those who have arrived by boat or plane and applied when onshore. The popular dominant discourse often refers to the latter group as the 'bad refugees', the alleged 'queue jumpers' who take the place of the 'good refugees' patiently waiting in refugee camps; however, we know that this is not the reality. Asylum seekers are demonised for paying traffickers and people smugglers for their journey, and more recently they are portrayed as 'terrorists' and a danger to society (Briskman 2021). The critiques highlight the controversial policy of Government that promotes offshore detention for asylum seekers in Australia (Mares 2016; Nipperess & Clark 2016; Boochani 2018; Fiske & Briskman 2020). The othering of refugees and asylum seekers detracts from addressing larger political human rights and social issues of exclusion and oppression, and increasingly climate change (Berchin et al. 2017) and needs to be seen as part of a globalised world (Castles & Miller 2009) with deep inequality.

Social Work: Health and Social Care

Immigration is a core area of public policy on which Australia depends for growth, employment and diversity (Neumann 2015). Social policy contributes to the delivery of services we identify as human services, public policy or welfare services. Implicit in understanding social policy is the Western concept of the welfare state, the origins of which were based in the religious orders of care and support. Both the church and the state have maintained an ideological separation between those seen as deserving and undeserving and this continues today with asylum seekers and refugees.

The critical social work literature points to the way neoliberalism contributes to the division between people in communities, the care of the sick who are considered blameless and therefore eligible for support, as compared to the poor who are seen as undeserving and treated more punitively (Garrett 2018; Gray & Webb 2013). This division has been referred to as the 'moral economy of care' and is seen to reflect 'wider societal values regarding the legitimate and illegitimate' use of resources and treatment of people (Watters 2007, p. 396). It is prominent and reflects an ideological tension, and indeed many now argue that there is an emergence of neo-welfare, characterised by privatisation of services, precarious employment of workers (the gig economy), and an increasing debt and surveillance of recipients (Garrett 2018, p. 205). Questions are also being asked about the role of social work in this space, particularly in perpetuating what McLaughlin described as:

> The tension between giving help without creating dependence, distinguishing between the 'deserving' and 'undeserving', assessing financial ability and familial and social networks has been, in one guise or another, a continual factor is social work and welfare to the present day.
>
> (McLaughlin, 2008, p. 5)

In Australia the activities of social workers involve working with a range of people, individually and collectively including older people, people with learning and physical disabilities, people with mental health difficulties, women, younger adults, or children. Much of the work in health care was developed in community health and community development models. The Community Health Movement of the late 1970s and 1980s reflected multi-disciplinary and multi-agency work in the community (Swerissen & Duckett 1997, p. 17). This emerged from social movements that promoted a human rights and equalities agenda and has since embraced an ecological perspective and one that acknowledges Indigenous practice and values (Ife 2016). In addition to this social work in hospital settings involves specialist work often with a range of professionals including psychologists, specialists in gerontology and child development. This approach to health care has tended to focus on the bio-medical model of physical illnesses, with treatment tending to conform to the Cartesian dualism of separating mind and body (Mehta 2011).

Social workers navigate these positions basing their decisions on ethical principles of access and equity, social justice, and human rights (Australian Association of Social Workers 2020). To empower and support culturally diverse community's social workers develop strategies to practice across micro, meso and macro levels. This involves navigating tensions that are prominent in community services with limited resources and addressing the diverse needs and rights of asylum seekers and refugees.

Trauma and Recovery Narratives

The experiences of refugees and asylum seekers are characterised by conditions of conflict, political upheaval, and economic instability. Many people have fled their homes in a state of emergency; they may have experienced torture, witnessed the death or loss of their family and communities, and lived in camps with limited protection and facilities. As Papadopoulos states, 'it is important to remember the obvious fact that becoming a refugee is not a psychological phenomenon per se; rather, it is exclusively a socio-political one, with psychological implications' (Papadopoulos 2007, p. 301).

Once people from refugee backgrounds arrive in a safe country their lives may be characterised by a complex set of circumstances including low income, poor housing, limited access to health care and social isolation. Studies have confirmed the negative impact on health that the asylum process has on those claiming asylum including the hostility they face from the host community (Coffey et al. 2010; Australian Human Rights Commission 2014; Hartley & Pedersen 2017). The field faces many challenges including obtaining accurate data on new arrivals (Correa-Velez & Gifford 2007; Jefferies, Ghezelbash & Hirsch 2020), identifying the specialist trauma needs of refugees and asylum seekers (Silove 2017), and specifying models of intervention and approaches to service provision that are effective for different groups of service users (Williams & Graham 2016). The needs of asylum seekers and refugees are heterogeneous and support services can build a sense of community and resilience. For example, Allwiess and Hilado (2018, pp. 46–51) emphasise housing affordability, access to a community, access to English language training, family and social support, financial and employment resources, and adequate health and mental health supports.

Although the emphasis on trauma and clinical mental health approaches have dominated the field (Bland, Renouf & Tullgren 2015), researchers and practitioners have highlighted other schools of thought that draw on trauma informed and community development models of participation (Ife 2016; Kenny & Connors 2017; Kaplan 2020). The identification and measurement of need is problematic in critical social work practice (Morley et al. 2019), and researchers have noted a shift in some services from considering need in terms of individual 'functioning', to more rights-based community, family based and child centred approaches (Mitchell & Correa-Velez 2010; Kaplan 2020). The emphasis on resilience and strength-based approaches have informed research and practice and promote cultural inclusivity, building social connections and 'normalises' the refugee experience (Marlowe 2010, 2018). This is an important aspect of social work practice and prompts us to think about how best to both include and respond to individuals, communities and different policy and practice.

Research has increasingly identified the arrival in the host country and the subsequent settlement period as having a major impact on the mental health and well-being of refugees and asylum seekers (Hartley & Pedersen 2017; Coffey et al. 2010; Allweiss & Hilado 2018). It highlights the challenges of providing mental health care, and how best to best provide trauma informed, culture informed and holistic services (Kaplan 2020). However, researchers have also emphasised that not all asylum seekers and refugees are traumatised 'victims', and assessment and care must respond to the needs of the individual. Critical social work theory can assist us to challenge individualist theories that can take away emphasis from structural factors (Morley et al. 2019). Importantly, practitioners have emphasised understanding the meaning of distress in a cultural context and recognising the way in which distress manifests as an appropriate reaction to grief, despair, and loss (Bogden & Marlow 2015; Williams & Graham 2016). Increasingly the literature with a focus on working with refugees and survivors of violence emphasises recovery models aimed at strengthening communities and supporting diversity (Allan 2014; Kaplan 2020).

Practice-Based Social Work Research in this Role and Field

How best to respond to the health and social care needs of asylum seekers and refugees often reflects the division between the medical and social models of health care, along with different theoretical approaches used in practice (Morley et al. 2019). There is evidence that three key determinants of mental health and well-being are social inclusion, freedom from discrimination and violence, and access to economic resources (Keleher and Armstrong 2005). A broad social model of public health considers the intersecting issues of class, race and gender, and how they impact on living environments, employment, education, and housing: all of which are vital for asylum seekers' and refugees' settlement.

Refugees and asylum seekers move between the two models of care - medical and social, often with restricted entitlements and limited status. Those working with asylum seekers and refugees often note how they fall outside standard social policy frameworks, and that this is an essential part of their professional role as advocates (Robinson 2014, 2020). Social workers who position themselves at a critical social work standpoint that incorporates anti-oppressive practice focus their efforts at three specific levels: the interpersonal, the cultural and the structural. Social work academics have described how this framework was developed by several theorists (see Dominelli 2017; Thompson 2021; Pease et al. 2016; Morley et al. 2019) and that it has the focus of ameliorating social injustice and oppression and promoting human rights. Working across these levels is important when dealing with the complexity of multiple systems and legislative frameworks such as immigration and forced migration. Let us consider an important issue that is current in many parts of the world.

Reflection: Responding to Communities during COVID-19 in 2020

In 2020 Melbourne's inner city public housing towers were closed due to COVID-19. Residents, many of whom are from refugee backgrounds and are front-line workers, were told to stay in their homes and 500 police surrounded their homes. Community leaders were not consulted, and many people were frightened and isolated. Food and medications were difficult to obtain, and children also had to stay indoors.

Reflection Questions

1 As a social worker what would you do?
2 Who would you involve and how might you go about this?
3 What are the key concerns for you about this situation and the approach of the Department of Health in taking this decision early in the pandemic?

Key Points: Working with Refugees

The legislative and procedural guidelines in Australia are complex and subject to frequent change and social workers are expected to understand how service users' claims may be affected. Key to working with asylum seekers and refugees is understanding how policy has impacted on them, particularly knowledge temporary protection measures and how these policies contribute to destitution and detention, and the treatment of unaccompanied asylum seeking children. For those people successful in obtaining refugees status social workers have a key role in the provision of settlement services and facilitating access to supports.

Settlement Services

The Humanitarian Settlement Program (HSP) provides a range of services which are defined as Immediate, Foundation, Specialised and Intensive Services (SIS). The HSP clearly states that the aim of the programme is to provide 'support to humanitarian entrants to build the skills and knowledge they need to become self-reliant and active members of the Australian community' (Australian Government 2021). Refugee Welcome Zones initiatives (RCOA 2020) have become part of many Australian cities, and the initiative sits within the wider global context of Welcoming Cities (UNESCO 2016), Sanctuary Cities (Mascareñas & Eitel 2019) and Solidarity Cities (Cristophe & Kron 2019). These aim to include refugees in a range of arts-and culture-based programmes, but also to build capacity within services and organisations to genuinely develop understanding of cultural diversity.

In Australia there is an active non-government and community sector works with refugees who are survivors of torture and trauma (Forum of Australian Services for Survivors of Torture and Trauma 2018; Kaplan 2020). Australia's network of torture and trauma services have advocated with newly arrived communities working in local councils and other community organisations, to establish pathways for people from refugee backgrounds in gaining accessible housing, health care, education, and employment.

There is extensive literature that highlights the key steps required for successful settlement that are both practical and theoretical (see Fozdar & Banki 2017; Marlowe 2018; Allweiss & Hilado 2018). Potocky and Naseh (2020) adopt a pancultural lens, highlighting universal human values affecting all of those affected by forced migration, noting how an intersectional point of view needs to be applied, including drawing on international law and policy. In Australia, successful programmes deliver a range of outcomes to young people in education from refugee backgrounds, and a State-wide network with a remit to provide training and development to a wide range of health and social care practitioners working with asylum seekers and refugees (Robinson 2020). However, the challenges facing communities often present as barriers to engagement with services as the following example illustrates.

Reflection: Settlement of New Arrivals

Between 2017 and 2019, over 100 Syrian and Syriac families were settled in Geelong in response to the Federal Government announcement that the number of refugees arriving in Australia would double from the intake of previous decades due to the war in Syria and Iraq (Australian Government 2019, p. 209). In a recent study of Syriac and Syrian refugees arriving in Geelong, regional Victoria, the community raised the concern of the lack of integration of services providing support and guidance in the initial stages of settlement (Robinson & Lamaro Haintz 2021).

While families were grateful for the opportunity of resettlement, many were frustrated. They described how, after the initial welcome from the host community, they found little ongoing support to assist them to integrate and establish themselves in the community. One man noted:

> But sometimes here, you've been for a month, you didn't see your case manager. And I've been – I faced this issue. It's closed weekends. I didn't know what to do. My Mum was very sick and I don't know where to go here. And then I talked with Agency later when we'd been part of the community. You have to give a plan for the client. A written plan. You will receive this service in this time. We will come on this day. You are free for three days. You can go where you want to go. But nothing changed. They hear and they don't do it.
>
> (Male 4; Focus group 1)

Reflection Questions

1. What types of issues would you as the social worker identify here that might inform decisions about how best to work with this group of new arrivals?
2. How would you address some of the concerns and issues in your practice?
3. Who would you involve and how might you go about this?

In Australia the system of *temporary protection visas* (TPVs, also called bridging visa E) for those who have been determined on Convention grounds to be refugees have been highly criticised (Mares 2016). This visa category provides temporary protection for three years, with the possibility of extension depending on the circumstances based on reassessment of the individual and the political situation of the country they were fleeing. It also prevents family re-unification which has had a great impact on the arrivals of asylum seekers from the Middle East. The implication for the applicant is that they are unable to settle and are anxious for the safety and well-being of their family. Mares (2016) notes 'Temporary protection is not policy as prevention, but policy as punishment' as it creates a 'marginalised and distraught cohort of people who live among us, but not with us' (pp. 191, 194).

Key Points: Working with Asylum Seekers

It was the Labour Government in Australia in the early 1990s that first initiated legislation to detain asylum seekers in remote camps while processing their immigration claims. Asylum seekers have less access rights to services and are currently in a combination of both offshore and on shore detention centres, and community-based detention (Sampson & Mitchell 2013, p. 102). Those in the community are reliant on voluntary community-based services and non-government organisations (NGOs). Australia has been unique in the world for introducing *mandatory detention* for all 'illegal' asylum seekers (those who enter without visas): despite claims that they are escaping persecution and therefore meet the UN Convention grounds for consideration (see United Nations High Commissioner for Refugees 2020). Commonwealth law enacted in 1994 and since has required:

> A person who does not hold a valid visa is an unlawful non-citizen and must be detained under the Migration Act 1958. Whether the person is placed in an immigration detention facility, or other arrangements are made, is determined using a risk-based approach.
>
> (Australia Border Force 2021)

Australia's policy of mandatory detention has become a highly divisive public policy issue. Considerable debate has ensued in Australia about the lawfulness of locking adults and children up, with limited course to appeal, and the role of services in detention (Coffey 2006; AHRC 2014; Briskman et al. 2012). Conflict has developed between and within political parties, with state and federal governments, between departments (such as immigration, education, and health), and of course, within the wider community.

There is a substantial body of research providing evidence of detainees with a demonstrated deterioration in their mental health (see von Werthern et al. 2018). One of the fundamental claims of those working with torture and trauma survivors is that they must feel safe to work towards recovery goals (Kaplan 2020). When in detention the person does not have support, activities, or freedom of choice to recuperate. Coffey has long argued that post-traumatic stress disorder is not treatable while the person is in detention, and the best clinicians can offer is possibly alleviating some symptoms and preventing further decline (Coffey 2006, p. 81). Practitioners, activists, and researchers have expressed concern regarding debates about political neutrality including the restrictions on them exposing the abuse and degrading treatment, and the dismissal of findings and policy that systematically violates human rights (Boochani 2018; Fleay et al. 2021; Field, Chung & Fleay 2021).

There is considerable literature from the community sector and academics documenting the barriers facing asylum seekers who are excluded from support and services, and the social workers working in this area of practice (Fiske & Briskman 2020; Hilado & Lundy 2018). Asylum seekers struggle to meet their basic needs when applying for asylum in Australia, and this has been exacerbated during the global pandemic as they are not eligible for any payments (RCOA 2021). Researchers describe limited access to Medicare, medication and medical equipment, a lack of work rights, income and housing, and a lengthy time waiting in uncertainty with a lack of support and advice (Field et al. 2021). The implications of these conditions are demonstrated to have a negative impact on mental health, and health overall and there is an on-going need for social workers to research and document these concerns and develop a strong evidence base with which to advocate for asylum seekers' rights.

The UNHCR defines an *unaccompanied asylum-seeking child* as being under 18 years old and not cared for by that child's usual carer. According to Convention on the Rights of the Child (General Comment no. 6, 2005):

> 'Unaccompanied children' (also called unaccompanied minors) are children, as defined in article 1 of the Convention, who have been separated from both parents and other relatives and are not being cared for by an adult who, by law or custom, is responsible for doing so.

In Australia there has been research and numerous reports documenting the detrimental effect of mandatory detention on children, and the ongoing developmental effects (Human Rights and Equal Opportunity Commission 2004; Australian Human Rights Commission 2014). Currently there are no arrivals of unaccompanied children in detention, but the legacy of this policy continues to impact young people and communities.

This section of the chapter has highlighted a range of challenging issues frontline workers deal with on a daily basis. The constant change involved in navigating the immigration system is both stressful and time consuming for frontline workers providing health and social care services. Another important area is the impact of the work on the frontline staff.

Support for Social Workers

The literature documents the stress of frontline workers who are placed in conflicted positions within and between services and working with service users who have high levels of anxiety and distress (Robinson 2014; Wirth et al. 2019; Posselt et al. 2020). Community organisations are known for demanding strong commitment from their workers, and many social workers have reported both trauma and stress because of exposure to the extreme hardship of their clients and communities, along with the organisational demands of the work (Robinson & Masocha 2017). These demands include rapid change in workplaces and increased performance measures and targets.

Increasingly frontline social workers supporting refugees and asylum seekers are often professionally and ethically compromised as they are confronted with dominant discourses that challenge a human rights-based approach (Briskman et al. 2012; Morley, Le & Briskman 2020). This is particularly the case for social workers who are subject to Section 41 of the Australian Border Force (ABF) Act 2015, which has secrecy and disclosure provisions. Challenging power dynamics in this charged political context can be extremely difficult and may result in the expulsion from organisations and/or criminal charges resulting in silencing of individuals and groups. Fiske and Briskman (2020) argue that social workers must adopt an anti-racist approach in their practice, policy and research in order to push back against institutional racism. It is important for social workers to demonstrate understanding of Australia's policies that violate international agreements it has signed such as the International Covenant on Civil and Political Rights (1976), the Convention Against Torture and the Convention on the Rights of the Child (1987) (see Human Rights Watch 2021).

For those working with people in distress, particularly those who had been in detention and suffered human rights abuses, supervision and peer support is essential. Research identifies that it is the shared responsibility of organisations to provide supervision and opportunities for support, along with the workers critical reflection that can contribute to staff retention, well-being, and a more positive experience of the work (Morley et al. 2020; Posselt et al. 2020). There is a need to nurture and support our colleagues and newly qualified social work staff to continue to work in this important sector.

Conclusion

Social workers are on the frontline of services working to address the complex issues for people subjected to immigration control and settlement in Australia. Research has focused on the importance of responding to the impact of pre migration experiences (including torture and trauma), the actual migratory journey, and post migration experience. There is a danger of treating all asylum seekers and refugees as the same, and not considering their individual and diverse experiences.

Embedded in social work practice is a tension between working to challenge policy approaches that are harmful to individuals, families and communities and working to address practical human needs. Social workers coming from a critical perspective need to imagine and advocate for different approaches to immigration. Strategies range from promoting change within organisations and the sector, doing advocacy work with other agencies and sectors to change policy, and conducting research with communities that promotes health and social care sensitive to the needs of refugees and asylum seekers. Hessle notes: 'Social workers are at the frontline of solidarity with vulnerable groups in all societies and international exchange of knowledge is necessary for dealing with transcultural problems' (Hessle 2007, p. 240). This involves challenging the legal frameworks governing the determination of immigration status, utilising participatory methods and strategies with service users and refugee communities to reflect their needs and concerns, and working with the broader community advocating for change in attitudes and government policy. It is rich and rewarding work, and social workers are well placed to engage in this demanding and expanding field.

Key Website Resources

Amnesty International Australia (www.amnesty.org.au).

The Australian Red Cross (www.redcross.org.au).

Asylum Seeker Resource Centre (ASRC), Melbourne (www.asrc.org.au).

Australian Human Rights Commission (www.humanrights.gov.au/our-work/asylum-seekers-and-refugees).

The Forum of Australian Services for Survivors of Torture and Trauma (http://fasstt.org.au).

International Detention Coalition (http://idcoalition.org).

National Council of Churches of Australia (www.ncca.org.au).

The Refugee Council of Australia (www.refugeecouncil.org.au).

Victorian Refugee Health Network (http://refugeehealthnetwork.org.au).

United Nations High Commissioner for Refugees (UNHCR) (www.unhcr.org) and Australia for UNHCR (www.unrefugees.org.au).

Note

1 The definition of a refugee has been defined by the UNHCR as 'owing to well-founded fear of being persecuted for reasons of race, religion, nationality, membership of a particular social

group or political opinion is outside the country of his nationality and is unable or, owing to such fear, is unwilling to avail himself of the protection of that country or to return there because there is a fear of persecution' (UNHCR 2020). Those seeking asylum and called 'asylum seekers' are seeking protection of this Convention. For the purposes of this chapter I will refer to both, making relevant distinctions as appropriate.

References

Allan, J. (2014). Reconciling the 'psycho-social/structural' in social work counselling with refugees. *British Journal of Social Work*, 45(6), 1699–1716.

Allweiss, S. and Hilado, A. (2018) The context of migration: pre-arrival, migration, and resettlment experiences. In Hilado, A. and Lundy, M. (eds), *Models for Practice with Immigrants and Refugees. Collaboration, Cultural Awareness, and Integrative Theory*. Thousand Oaks, CA: Sage.

Australian Association of Social Workers. (2020) Code of ethics. Retrieved from www.aasw.asn.au/practitioner-resources/code-of-ethics.

Australian Border Force. (2021) Australian immigration detention. Retrieved from www.abf.gov.au/about-us/what-we-do/border-protection/immigration-detention.

Australian Government. (2019). Department of Immigration and Border Protection annual report 2018–2019. Retrieved from www.homeaffairs.gov.au/reports-and-pubs/Annualreports/home-affairs-annual-report-2018-19.pdf.

Australian Government. (2021) Humanitarian Settlement Program (HSP). Retrieved from https://immi.homeaffairs.gov.au/settling-in-australia/humanitarian-settlement-program.

Australian Human Rights Commission. (2014). The forgotten children: national inquiry into children in immigration detention. Retrieved from www.humanrights.gov.au/our-work/asylum-seekers-and-refugees/national-inquiry-children-immigration-detention-2014.

Australian Human Rights Commission. (2021) Management of COVID-19 risks in immigration detention. Retrieved from https://humanrights.gov.au/our-work/asylum-seekers-and-refugees/publications/management-covid-19-risks-immigration-detention.

Berchin, I. I., Valduga, I. B., Garcia, J. & de Andrade, J. B. S. O. (2017) Climate change and forced migrations: an effort towards recognizing climate refugees. *Geoforum*, 84, 147–150.

Beddoe L. (2010) Surveillance or reflection: professional supervision in 'the risk society'. *British Journal of Social Work*, 40(4), 1279–1296.

Bhabha, J. & Crock, M. (2007) *Seeking Asylum Alone: Unaccompanied and Separated Children and Refugee Protection in Australia, the UK and the US*. Sydney: Themis Press.

Bogden, R. & Marlowe, J. (2015) Asylum discourse in New Zealand: moral panic and a culture of indifference. *Australian Social Work*, 70(1), 104–115.

Boochani, B. (2018) *No Friend but the Mountains: Writing from Manus Prison*. Picador Australia.

Bland, R., Renouf, N. & Tullgren, A. (2015) *Social Work Practice in Mental Health. An Introduction*. Allen and Unwin.

Briskman, L. (2021) Racialised citizenship: challenging the Australian imaginary. In Weber, L. and Tazreiter, C. (eds.), *Edward Elgar Handbook of Migration and Global Justice*. Cheltenham: Edward Elgar Publishing.

Briskman, L., Zion, D. and Loff, B. (2012) Care or collusion in asylum seeker detention. *Ethics and Social Welfare*, 6(1), 37–55.

Castles, S. & Miller, M. J. (2009) *The Age of Migration: International Population Movements in the Modern World*. Palgrave Macmillan.

Coffey, G. (2006). Locked Up Without Guilt or Sin: The Ethics of Mental Health Service Delivery in Immigration Detention. *Psychiatry, Psychology and Law*, 13(1), 67–90.

Coffey, G. J., Kaplan, I., Sampson, R. C. & Tucci, M. M. (2010). The meaning and mental health consequences of long-term immigration detention for people seeking asylum. *Social Science and Medicine*, 70(12), 2070–2079.

Correa-Velez, I. & Gifford, S. M. (2007). When the right to be counted doesn't count: The politics and challenges of researching the health of asylum seekers. *Critical Public Health*, 17(3), 273–281.

Cristophe, W. & Kron, S. (eds). (2019). Solidarity cities in Europe charity or pathways to citizenship: a new urban policy approach. Retrieved from www.rosalux.de/en/publication/id/41319/solidarity-cities-in-europe?cHash=36be577ba1c636e9bf9f6ede61b4f1e6.

Dominelli, L. (2017). *Anti-Racist Social Work* (4th edition). Macmillan International Higher Education.

Field, R. S., Chung, D. & Fleay, C. (2021) Working with restrictions: A scoping review of social work and human service practice with people seeking asylum in the Global North. *The British Journal of Social Work*, 51(1), 57–76.

Fiske, L. & Briskman, L., (2020). Transcending racism in asylum politics: Quest for social workers. In Singh, G. and Masocha, S. (eds), *Anti-racist Social Work: International Perspectives*. Red Globe Press.

Fleay, C., Kenny, M.A., Andaveh, A., Askari, S., Hassani, R., Leaney, K. & Lee, T. (2021). Doing something for the future: building relationships and hope through refugee and asylum seeker advocacy in Australia. In *Handbook of Migration and Global Justice*. Edward Elgar Publishing.

Fook, J. (2016) *Social Work: A Critical Approach to Practice* (3rd edition). Sage.

Forum of Australian Services for Survivors of Torture and Trauma. (2018). Never turning away: Australia's world leading program of assistance for survivors of torture and trauma (FASTT). Retrieved from https://fasstt.org.au/wordpress/wp-content/uploads/2018/12/FASSTT_BOOKLET_2017_A4_FA_web.pdf.

Fozdar, F. & Banki, S. (2017) Settling refugees in Australia: achievements and challenges. *International Journal of Migration and Border Studies*, 3(1), 43–66.

Garrett, P.M., (2018) *Welfare Words: Critical Social Work & Social Policy*. Sage.

Gray, M. & Webb, S. A. (eds) (2013) *The New Politics of Social work*. Palgrave Macmillan.

Hartley, L. K. & Pedersen, A. (2017). Asylum seekers and resettled refugees in Australia: Predicting social policy support prejudice versus emotion. *Journal of Social and Political Psychology*, 3(1), 179–197.

Hessle, S. (2007) Globalisation: implications for international development work, social work and the integration of immigrants in Sweden. In Dominelli, L. (ed.), *Revitalising Communities in a Globalising World*. Farnham: Ashgate.

Hilado, A. & Lundy, M. (2018). *Models for Practice with Immigrants and Refugees. Collaboration, Cultural Awareness, and Integrative Theory*. Thousand Oaks, CA: Sage.

Human Rights and Equal Opportunity Commission. (2004) *A Last Resort? National Inquiry into Children in Immigration Detention*. Human Rights and Equal Opportunity Commission.

Human Rights Watch. (2021) *Australia: Address Abuses Raised at UN Review. Countries Criticize Failures on Refugees, Children, Indigenous Rights*. Human Rights Watch. Retrieved from www.hrw.org/news/2021/01/21/australia-address-abuses-raised-un-review.

Ife, J. (2016) *Community Development in an Uncertain World*. Vision, analysis and practice. (2nd edn) Cambridge University Press.

Jefferies, R., Ghezelbash, D. & Hirsch, A. (2020). Assessing refugee protection claims at Australian airports: the gap between law, policy, and practice. *Melbourne University Law Review*, 44(1), 162–211.

Kaplan, I. (2020) *Rebuilding Shattered Lives. Integrated Trauma Recovery for People from Refugee Backgrounds*. Victorian Foundation for Survivors of Torture.

Keleher, H. & Armstrong, R. (2005) *Evidence-Based Mental Health Promotion Resource*. Melbourne: Public Health Group, Victorian Department of Human Services.

Kenny, S. & Connors, P. (2017) *Developing Communities for the Future* (5th edition). Cengage.

McLaughlin, K. (2008) *Social Work, Politics and Society: From Radicalism to Orthodoxy*. Bristol: Policy Press.

Mares, P. (2016) *Not Quite Australian. How Temporary Migration is Changing the Nation*. The Text Publishing Company.

Marlowe, J. M. (2010) Beyond the discourse of trauma: shifting the focus on Sudanese refugees. *Journal of Refugee Studies* 23(2), 183–198.

Marlowe, J. (2018) *Belonging and Transnational Refugee Settlement: Unsettling the Everyday and Extraordinary*. Routledge.

Mascareñas, B. & Eitel, K. (2019) Sanctuary cities: a global perspective. Retrieved from www.cidob.org/en/articulos/anuario_internacional_cidob/2019/sanctuary_cities_a_global_perspective.

Mehta, N. (2011) Mind-body dualism: a critique from a health perspective. *Mens Sana Monographs*, 9(1), 202.

Morley, C., Ablett, P. & Macfarlane, S. (2019) *Engaging with Social Work: A Critical Introduction*. Cambridge University Press.

Morley, C., Le, C. & Briskman, L. (2020) The role of critical social work education in improving ethical practice with refugees and asylum seekers, *Social Work Education*, 39:4, 403–416.

Mitchell, J. & Correa-Velez, I. (2010). Community development with survivors of torture and trauma: an evaluation framework. *Community Development Journal*, 45(1), 90–110.

Neumann, K. (2015) *Across the Seas: Australia's Response to Refugees: A History*. Black Inc.

Nipperess, S. & Clark, S. (2016) Anti-oppressive practice with people seeking asylum in Australia: reflections from the field. In Pease, B., Goldingay, S., Hosken, N. and Nipperess, S. (eds), *Doing Critical Social Work: Transformative Practices for Social Justice*. Allen and Unwin.

Nipperess, S. & Williams, C. (2019) *Critical Multicultural Practice in Social Work: New Perspectives and Practices*. (223–239). Allen and Unwin.

Papadopoulos, R. (2007) Refugees, trauma and adversity-activated development. *European Journal of Psychotherapeutic Counselling*, 9(3), 301–312.

Pease, B., Goldingay, S., Hoskin, N. and Nipperness, S. (2016) *Doing Critical Social Work. Transformative Practices for Social Justice*. Allen and Unwin.

Posselt, M., Baker, A., Deans, C. and Procter, N. (2020) Fostering mental health and well-being among workers who support refugees and asylum seekers in the Australian context. *Health & Social Care in the Community*, 28(5), 1658–1670.

Potocky, M. & Naseh, M., (2020) *Best Practices for Social Work with Refugees and Immigrants*. Columbia University Press.

Refugee Council of Australia. (2020) Refugee welcome zones. Retrieved from www.refugeecouncil.org.au/refugee-welcome-zones/.

Refugee Council of Australia. (2021) Information about social security and COVID-19. Retrieved from www.refugeecouncil.org.au/social_security_faq_covid-19/.

Robinson, K. (2014) Voices from the Front Line: Social Work with Refugees and Asylum Seekers in Australia and the UK, *British Journal of Social Work*, vol. 44, no. 6, pp. 1602–1620.

Robinson, K. (2020) A 'good news' story of social inclusion: refugee resettlement in Australia. In Crisp, B. A. and Takert, A. (eds) *Sustaining Social Inclusion* (pp. 231–244). Routledge.

Robinson, K. & Masocha, S. (2017) Divergent practices in statutory and voluntary-sector settings? Social work with asylum seekers. *British Journal of Social Work*, 47(5), 1517–1533.

Robinson, K. & Lamaro Haintz, G. (2021) Is anyone listening to us? 'They're given feedback and there's no outcomes': Settlement for newly arrived Syrians in regional Australia. *Ethics and Social Welfare*, online ahead of print.

Sampson, R. and Mitchell, G. (2013) Global trends in immigration detention and alternatives to detention: practical, political and symbolic rationales. *Journal on Migration and Human Security*, 1(3), 97–121.

Silove, D. (2017) Effective interventions and models for refugee trauma. *Refugee Transitions*, 32, 34–39.

Swerissen, H. & Duckett, S. (1997) Health policy and financing. In H. Gardner (ed.), *Health Policy in Australia*. Oxford: Oxford University Press.

Thompson, N. (2021). *Anti-Discriminatory Practice: Equality, Diversity and Social Justice*. Bloomsbury Publishing.

UNESCO. (2016) *Welcoming Refugees and Migrants: Enhancing Effective Urban Governance in an Age of Migration*. UNESCO. Retrieved from www.refworld.org/pdfid/5a5f429a4.pdf.

United Nations High Commissioner for Refugees. (2020) *UNHCR Global Report 2020*. United Nations High Commissioner for Refugees. Retrieved from www.unhcr.org/en-au/the-global-report.html.

von Werthern, M., Robjant, K., Chui, Z., Schon, R., Ottisova, L., Mason, C. & Katona, C. (2018). The impact of immigration detention on mental health: a systematic review. *BMC Psychiatry*, 18(1), 1–19.

Watters, C. (2007) Refugees at Europe's borders: the moral economy of care, *Transcultural Psychiatry*, 44, 394–417.

Williams, C. and Graham, M. J. (2016) *Social Work in a Diverse Society. Transformative Practice with Black and Minority Ethnic Individuals and Communities*. Policy Press.

Wirth, T., Mette, J., Prill, J., Harth, V. & Nienhaus, A., (2019) Working conditions, mental health and coping of staff in social work with refugees and homeless individuals: a scoping review. *Health & Social Care in the Community*, 27(4), e257–e269.

15 Health Social Work in Regional, Rural and Remote Settings

Responding to the Intersection of Location, Disadvantaged Populations and Communities

Ros Darracott, Niki Edwards and Julie King

Introduction

The highly dispersed nature of much of Australia's population has required development of a breadth of health care delivery models in regional, rural, and remote communities (Darracott & Lonne, 2017). While there is substantial variation, overall, citizens living outside of major cities experience poorer health outcomes than their metropolitan counterparts and are disadvantaged across the socio-economic indices in regard to health, education, housing, and finance (Alston, 2015). Climate change poses additional challenges with increased natural disasters (including pandemics), and rising temperatures.

This chapter examines experiences of Australians living in regional, rural, and remote communities where distance, drought, climate change, workforce challenges and the nexus of social, health, economic, and environmental policy influences health social work practice. Geographical disadvantage is explored with particular attention on the intersection of structural oppressions, including the experiences of Aboriginal and Torres Strait Islander peoples, people with disability, people from refugee and migrant backgrounds, people where English is another language, and older people. The chapter argues that health social work practice must be culturally safe, adopt a climate aware lens, be contextualised, creative, and community-embedded in order to respond to the unique challenges and strengths of Australians living outside major cities.

One size does *not* fit all in Australian health social work and this is particularly relevant to regional, rural, and remote practice given the diversity of the Australian people and the locations they live in (Rural Health Standing Committee, 2011). The nature of Australia's population dispersion, climate and terrain, history of colonisation, unique health issues, wellbeing of communities, and economic and social diversity, leads to the need for an array of service delivery models and responses to achieve a semblance of adequate health service accessibility. Health services must be contextualised to be successful (Wakerman & Humphreys, 2011, p. 118); and health social work practice also needs to adapt to the unique dynamics and needs of the particular community/ies served.

Conceptual Framework: 'Person as Place'

The profession of social work plays a pivotal social change role in society; with ethical and moral obligations for promotion of human rights, social justice and inclusive social structures that result in better living environments for all citizens (Rambaree, 2020). Nonetheless, social work has been heavily critiqued in recent years for overlooking the intertwined nature of social and environmental justice; and in particular a failure to

DOI: 10.4324/9781003330745-18

affirm the importance of the physical environment, environmental justice, and care for planet earth (Dominelli, 2013). Indigenous social work and rural social work (which is heavily influenced by Indigenous social work) are the two fields of social work practice that have long embraced a holistic understanding of people and their natural and physical environments (Zapf, 2009). While 'person-in-environment' or 'person: environment' is well-established as the foundational metaphor of the social work profession, the *social* environment has been privileged and the physical and natural environment systematically overlooked in the application of that metaphor by mainstream social work (Zapf, 2009). A significant shift in the interest social work pays to the natural and physical environment is underway with the rise of green or eco-social work perspectives and practices (see for example Boetto, 2019; Dominelli, 2012). However, the privileging of the social environment is now firmly entrenched and somewhat cemented into the profession's persona.

'People as place' is proposed by Zapf (2009) as a new foundational metaphor for social work; and this strongly resonates with rural and remote social work practice. As a metaphor it shifts the focus from the individual (person) to the community (people); addresses the separation of people from their environment by the use of the term *as* rather than 'in' or 'and'; and replaces the term environment, which while not problematic in itself, has become wedded to an interpretation of 'social environment', moving thinking to *place* which carries none of that baggage (Zapf, 2009). Further, Zapf (2009) argues that such a metaphor lends itself to a professional purpose of 'Living well in place', allowing a critical social work lens to be more easily integrated.

While 'people as place' would serve all fields of practice well as a foundational metaphor, at the very least, for health social workers in regional, rural, and remote practice, it provides a solid base from which to understand and integrate the breadth of knowledges, skills, and approaches required. The professional purpose of 'living well in place' is especially relevant for health practice in these contexts where the health and wellbeing of the *people* is so dependent on the health of the *place*; and in a field where the people worked with often experience dislocation from their place simply to access ongoing health treatment and essential services. This chapter purposefully embraces and invites readers to approach health social work in non-metropolitan places, from this important perspective.

Understanding the Context

Approximately 71% of Australia's population lives in major cities along the coastline with the remaining 29% living in highly dispersed settlements in the regional and more remote areas of the country (Australian Institute of Health and Welfare, 2018). 'Regional', 'rural', and 'remote' are not discrete, easily defined categories occupied by homogenous communities. There is a multiplicity of definitions of what constitutes each category with some population based, others distance based, and access based also used. Health service planning is based on degrees of 'remoteness' and uses categories of 'major cities', 'inner regional', 'outer regional', 'remote' and 'very remote'. These categories, developed by the Australian Bureau of Statistics, consider distances people have to travel to access essential services (Australian Bureau of Statistics, 2018). Distance, however, does not equal access; consider the differences between a well-maintained bitumen road and a black soil road in the rain or a daily versus twice-weekly public bus service. While the categories are clearly problematic, what is more important for social workers to understand is that a label and one axis of measurement is not enough to understand a place or the experience of that place.

Social construction is very much at play with particular relevance to the simplistic binary of 'rural' or 'remote'. Whether or not a place *feels* regional, rural, or remote (or very remote for that matter) depends on individual perception and that perception can change over time and circumstance or be related to access to resources (Roberts & Guenther, 2021). With good community networks and reliable access to resources and transport, quite geographically distant places may be experienced simply as non-urban without deficits attached. Defining 'rural' or 'urban' is a socio-political activity which, while somewhat based on location and terrain, is heavily influenced by power dynamics and dominant discourses that default urban as 'normal' (Malatzky & Bourke, 2016). The use of the term 'non-metropolitan', while more expedient than 'regional, rural, and remote', exemplifies this positioning of urban as central and 'normal' (Alston, 2015). It is important social workers are aware of the urban norm from which all else is measured; value people, place, and community rather than conceptualising non-urban environments as problems to be solved (Roberts & Green, 2013; Roberts & Guenther, 2021). Complexity is a growing concern and challenge for social workers in contemporary practice and working in non-urbanised environments poses specific challenges (Harvey & Jones, 2021).

While constructions of regional, rural, and remote are contested and slippery, there is also no such thing as a singular 'rural culture'. Rather than a singular 'rural culture' it is more useful to consider how meaning is constructed in a particular place; for examples through consideration of the economic base, power dynamics, and historical events that enable particular discourses to emerge and dominate (Wendt, 2009). The culture of a place is fluid and ever evolving; and while influenced by broader societal discourses and structures there is no uniform way this is constructed and experienced across communities.

Framework for Regional, Rural and Remote Health

A useful framework for understanding rural and remote health is provided by Bourke, Humphreys, Wakerman and Taylor (2012) and arguably has application in regional centres as well. The framework captures how important context is to both the shaping of a community's health and how, in response, it should shape health practice. It links the micro, meso and macro factors influencing health and health behaviour. The approach to power that underpins the framework (Gidden's structuration theory) recognises while that power is exercised through the structures that guide our work and society more broadly (for example, policies and role descriptions), we have agency in the way we interpret and act on these structures and in turn can influence the shape of those structures. Some structures are enabling, others are constraining. In this way we, and others, actively shape the health and health services of the communities in which we work. The framework has six key concepts: 'geographical isolation; the rural locale, health responses in the rural locales; broader health systems; broader social structures; and power relations at all levels' (Bourke et al., 2012, p. 498).

Geographical isolation: the geographical location of someone experiencing a health issue has concrete and pragmatic ramifications (Bourke et al., 2012). A diagnosis of acute kidney disease for someone living in a major city is experienced and managed very differently to the same health event occurring in someone living in a town with a population of 100 and no formal health services.

The rural locale: refers to not just the place (the natural and built environment) in which the person lives but the unique dynamics or social relations of *that* place. The power dynamics of the community, access to resources, social connectedness (or not), information flow – all of the elements of a community of place – influence health outcomes in that place. Those social relations, power and resource dynamics influence health behaviours which in turn influence health needs, health status, and health outcomes (Bourke et al., 2012).

Health responses in rural locales: includes the formal and informal health responses that are performed in the rural locale. This includes the full range of health services that might be established but it is the 'how' rather than the 'what' that is of most interest in this sphere. This is where those in the community and those working in the health system can shape and influence service responses and consequently shape health; where they can be responsive to the unique dynamics of their particular community, be innovative, and contextually sensitive – or not. For example, the local chamber of commerce may go into partnership with the state health service to seek innovative ways of supporting the availability of allied health services to the community (Bourke et al., 2012). For social workers employed in these health services this is where agency can be exercised, and practice can be community-embedded rather than the community being 'done to'. Community-embedded practice takes the time to know the community in all its diversity, works respectfully with local values, and strengthens rather than undermines key natural support networks and processes (Cheers, Darracott & Lonne, 2007; Darracott & Lonne, 2017). This sphere is of course influenced by the 'broader health systems' and 'broader social structures' but, if seeking to be contextually responsive, it would not be dictated to by these and simply reproduce unjust power relations.

Broader health systems: refers to the interplay between key stakeholder health systems. Our health systems are influenced by State and Federal health policies, funding arrangements, the dual system of private and public health, professional bodies (such as the Australian Medical Association and Australian Association of Social Workers), trade unions, and political debates regarding state versus federal responsibility. These health systems can promote or constrain innovation and contextual responsiveness (Bourke et al., 2012). As social workers, it is imperative that we understand this sphere so that we recognise opportunities when they arise.

Broader social structures: this sphere recognises the broader structures in society that serve to privilege some and oppress others and that create poor outcomes in terms of the social determinants of health. These structural issues all play a part in impacting the health of the individual in the rural locale (Bourke et al., 2012). Consider the structures that promote Western ideas of health and medicine over Indigenous understandings and approaches; that promote economic growth over environmental protection; and that promote urban-centric perspectives and health economics as a foundation for rural health services over socially and environmentally just approaches. How we practice, and whether we simply reproduce and reinforce the inequities generated at the structural and systems levels, depends on the agency exercised in practice. This approach to understanding how it is that regional, rural, and remote health is manifested and maintained helps social workers to avoid perpetuating a deficit and pathologised narrative of practice outside of urban communities.

Implications of Population Dispersion and Negative Constructions of 'Remoteness' on Health Service Delivery

While the challenges facing rural and remote communities are real, it would seem that the work done to draw attention to the health challenges in rural and remote practice has had some unintended consequences. Raising political and community awareness has been essential in garnering support for innovative responses and resourcing; however, it also reinforces a long-standing deficit discourse of rural and remote communities and health practice. This further adds to recruitment and retention issues in the health workforce, thus exacerbating health problems (Malatzky & Bourke, 2018; Wakerman et al., 2019). There is evidence of geographical narcissism (Fors, 2018) where dominant societal narratives of the city being 'progressive' and rural and remote areas being 'backwards' and disadvantaged result in incorrect assumptions around homogenous communities. The diversity and richness of the different experiences can be overlooked. It also takes an urban-centric view where urban becomes the 'norm' to which all else is compared. Narratives regarding high workloads and burnout have been privileged over the richness of practice that comes with an extended scope; which is further exacerbated by an increased valuing of 'specialism' (often accompanied by prestige and increased pay) over generalism (Malatzky & Bourke, 2016, 2018).

The deficit discourse of rural health, and hence non-metropolitan practice, is generated by comparing rural health outcomes to urban outcomes: although these are hardly comparable given the disparity in access to essential services. It could be argued that there are clearly many strengths for rural health outcomes to be as good as they are given the resources they have at their disposal (Malatzky & Bourke, 2016). While the Australian Institute of Health and Welfare clearly note the health disparities between non-metropolitan areas and major cities, the HILDA (Household, Income and Labour Dynamics in Australia) report notes that life satisfaction, community connectedness, and participation are higher for those living in non-metropolitan areas (AIHW, 2019). While there are personal, professional, and practical challenges associated with working in rural health settings, there are also advantages and benefits, including variety in work, autonomy of practice and the feeling that one is doing an important job (Campbell, McAllister & Eley, 2012).

Negative discourses aside, the dispersed nature of Australia's population leads to some very practical problems in service delivery. *Critical mass* is an important concept in service planning that is not often explicitly discussed in urban settings where it more easily achieved. Critical mass refers to the number of people required to be in need of a service to make delivery of that service viable in both an economic and workforce sense (Darracott & Lonne, 2017; Russell & Humphreys, 2016). Applied in the health context, this leads to the current tiered system of service delivery. There are some specialist health services that are only available in the major cities because there is not the critical mass of potential patients and specialist workforce to sustain such services in areas with lower populations (OECD, 2016). Regional cities now offer a broad array of tertiary health services providing somewhat more accessible services for the majority of health conditions; whereas health services in smaller communities tend to be more primary health care focused with acute or emergency conditions being stabilised and transferred to the closest community with the required service level. Discrete primary health care services (similar to urban general practice clinics) work well in more closely settled communities and as the population becomes more dispersed the use of 'hub and spoke' outreach models and fly-in/fly-out or virtual clinics becomes more prevalent (Wakerman et al., 2008; Wakerman & Humphreys, 2011). These more innovative approaches to health care can be quite successful if they are suitably supported by adequate resourcing, policy at both State and Commonwealth levels, strong governance and leadership, and have community support (Wakerman & Humphreys, 2011).

Telehealth has been held up as an important strategy for improving health service access (Bradford, Caffery & Smith, 2016). Regardless, one of the challenges of visiting and tele-health services is the lack of contextual knowledge held by the service providers. Social workers have a key role in ensuring that visiting or tele-health services (such as an Aged Care Assessment) are provided with adequate context to ensure an appropriate assessment can be made (Darracott & Lonne, 2017). Social workers who provide visiting services themselves need to strive to ensure that their practice in the recipient community is community-embedded – which requires building strong community networks (Cheers et al., 2007; Darracott & Lonne, 2017). The Australian Association of Social Workers (AASW) has published guidance on the delivery of telehealth services for social workers (particularly under Medicare Better Outcomes) that aims to assist practitioners to enable provision of safe and effective consultations and outlines the administrative and technical considerations when introducing this mode of service delivery (AASW, 2020).

Consequently, social work practice in a tertiary hospital or community health service delivered in a major city can look and feel quite different to social work services in an outer regional area. In a major city or even in the regional hospitals, the social worker is likely to be part of a large team and may work in quite specialised areas such as traumatic brain injury; or be focused on one area of presentation, such as the Emergency Department. Whereas the social worker in a rural hospital may be in a small team, or be a sole practitioner, working across the whole hospital. Depending on how dispersed the communities are and how dense the population is, the hospital social worker may also be the community health social worker and/or may cover a large geographical area comprised of several small hospitals and out-patient clinics. The hub and spoke model is a common model in Australia where a hub of health services is located in larger town, with outreach services (usually a mix of face-to-face and telehealth) being provided to the smaller towns in the service region (Wakerman & Humphreys, 2011). Because of Australia's highly dispersed population, the service regions tend to be very large. On the spectrum of specialised to generalised social work services, the more remote the location the more generalist and generic the service delivery tends to be.

Reflection: Mr Johnson's Story

Mr Johnson is 75 years old and lives by himself on a small working farm about 45 minutes drive from a regional city. He is well connected to his neighbours and they are aware he has been in hospital after having had a stroke. Mr Johnson now requires a four-wheel walker for mobility, has reduced hearing and is ready for discharge.

Reflection Questions

What might need to be considered when planning with Mr Johnson for his discharge? What additional information would need to be considered if the temperature is 39 degrees Celsius, with a high bushfire danger in his area?

The Lived Experience of Health Services

People living in non-metropolitan locations experience disadvantages associated with urban-centric policy development and resource distribution that often intersect with other experiences of marginalisation and disadvantage related to cultural identity, class, language, disability, age, sexual orientation, gender identity, sex, and visa status (Robards et al.,

2020). Despite the stereotypes, non-metropolitan communities are diverse places with people who are far from homogenous. Intersectionality draws attention to the multiplicity of people's identities and how processes of oppression and privilege intersect in quite unique ways as opposed to being simply additive or hierarchical (Pease, 2013).

Some communities are more inclusive of particular groups of people whereas some are othering. Importantly, inclusivity of one group does not necessarily mean inclusivity of another; hence, social workers need to take time to understand the dynamics of individual communities. For example, inclusivity of difference may be dependent on whether a person in a community is considered an 'insider' or 'outsider' (Heslop, Burns & Lobo, 2018). Difference may be accepted for the insider but not for the outsider or vice versa. Advocacy and challenging dominant narratives that foster discrimination are key social work roles across all fields of practice. It may be imperative for health social workers given access to specialised services is impacted by critical mass. For example, depending on the size and location of the community, access to specialist LGBTIQ+ services or refugee and migrant services can be very difficult (Darracott & Lonne, 2017).

It is also imperative that health social workers embrace a cultural safety lens. Cultural safety has been defined as the individual and institutional knowledge, skills, attitudes and capabilities needed to deliver optimal health care for Aboriginal and Torres Strait Islander peoples as determined by First Nations individuals, families and communities (Cox, Taua, Drummond & Kidd, 2020). It is imperative that health social workers use a cultural safety lens that understands it is *the patient* who identifies they are experiencing culturally safe practice; hence, social workers must critically reflect on not only their contributions but also their profession's role in colonisation (Fleming, Creedy & West, 2020).

Cultural safety embraces a broad definition of culture that is not limited to age, disability and impairment experiences, diverse gender identities, employment or occupational status, ethnic background including refugee or migrant experiences, or religious and spiritual beliefs; and recognises the intersectionality of these experiences. Consequently, it has direct relevance to work with all people experiencing oppression (Cox et al., 2020). Being culturally safe obliges health social workers to recognise the dynamic and intersectional nature of 'culture' and the nexus with rural or remote location through critical reflection and reflexivity.

Aboriginal and Torres Strait Islander Peoples

Cultural safety necessitates examination of the impacts of colonisation, intergenerational trauma and the privileging of Western white ways of knowing and doing in Australia's health systems that continues to have serious implications for the health of Aboriginal and Torres Strait Islander peoples and communities (Duthie, 2019). Chapter 12 examines these critical issues; however, it is important to note the strong intersection with rural and remote health. The 2016 census data shows that while more First Nations Australians live in major cities (33%) or inner regional areas (24%) than elsewhere in the country, the proportion of Indigenous Australians to non-Indigenous Australians in remote and very remote communities is higher (ABS, 2018). That is, in major cities Indigenous Australians comprise 1.7% of the population and 4.4% of the population in inner regional areas; whereas this grows to 7.9% of the outer regional population, 18% of the remote population, and 47% of the very remote population (ABS, 2018). Thus, the ongoing health disadvantages experienced in remote and very remote communities are intertwined with the health disadvantages related to colonisation and systemic racism. Trauma-informed practice is critical to Indigenous healing and should be implemented by health social workers to enable cultural safety (Tujague & Ryan, 2021).

Reflection: Practice in the Rural Locale

In one small town of 1500 people with a history of colonisation that had fractured relationships between Aboriginal nations and created class-based fractures in the non-Indigenous community, the social worker needed to find a way to make their service accessible to as many people as possible – they were the only social work service that visited the community. Community fractures had led to a lack of trust in many agencies across family, class, and racial divides that meant that no single agency was seen as safe and trustworthy. By working from a number of agencies, as well as offering home and park visits, and developing credible relationships across these divisions, the health social worker enabled service accessibility across the community.

Poverty and Unemployment

While educational attainment levels and employment rates are lower outside of the major cities (Australian Institute of Health and Welfare, 2018), this is somewhat symptomatic of urban and euro-centric policy development that limits access to education and employment opportunities (Commonwealth of Australia, 2020; Prout, 2008). Consequently, there are lower income levels (National Rural Health Alliance, 2014). Unemployment is not the only driver of poverty as there is also a significant problem of low-income employment and under-employment. Adding to the financial burden is the higher cost of living experienced in rural and remote areas with food costs being 10–20% higher and fuel 10% higher than urban areas (National Rural Health Alliance, 2014; Whelan et al., 2018). Lower income, in turn, contributes to poor health outcomes and lower engagement with health services (despite poor health) because of the cost of access. An ageing population and higher retiree rate outside of the major cities also contributes to lower income levels (Australian Institute of Health and Welfare, 2018). The higher costs of food, fuel, travel to health and education all compound the issue of lower incomes (National Rural Health Alliance, 2014).

Disability

Australians living in rural and remote areas experience higher levels of illness, injury and disability than the urban population, yet have limited access to quality services (Bohanna et al., 2021). For people with disabilities in rural and remote communities, their experience of services all too often involves little continuity of care and harrowing transitions between services and life stages. Communities, families, and informal carers often shoulder an enormous burden of care without recognition, payment, or support (Hussain, Wark & Ryan, 2018). While there is a specific chapter on the needs of people living with disability (see Chapter 10), it is important for health social workers to recognise that disability further amplifies disadvantages experienced in non-urban areas due to challenges in accessing appropriate health care and supports. The National Disability Insurance Scheme (NDIS) has included a rural and remote strategy, however despite this, it appears that the NDIS has struggled to deliver high-quality person-centred services to rural and remote communities due to thin markets (few providers) and socio-economic disadvantaged communities (Hussain et al., 2018). Health social work in this space may require legal liaison and advocacy to ensure rights are met.

Climate Change and Health Social Work Practice in Regional, Rural and Remote Australia

Climate change is a major concern for Australians but regional, rural, and remote communities experience significant risk. These communities are often directly dependent upon primary industries (farming, grazing, fishing, forestry) which are particularly vulnerable to droughts, floods, fires, cyclones, and unpredictable weather patterns. Risks associated with displacement are especially concerning for First Nations people (Altman & Jordan, 2018). Disasters destroy infrastructure and access to already scarce services can be disrupted for long periods (Verrinder & Talbot, 2015). The economic restructuring of the primary industries in recent decades have left them and the communities dependent on them with very little economic resilience. Other economic activities such as tourism can also be disrupted for extended periods of time. Adopting adaptation strategies becomes more challenging with increased remoteness due to the pre-existing infrastructure problems of access, housing, water quality, and health services (Verrinder & Talbot, 2015). Remote First Nations communities are particularly vulnerable for these reasons.

Climate vulnerability needs to be considered a serious issue for health and wellbeing given it is intertwined with social and health vulnerability; specifically exacerbating pre-existing inequalities in the health system (Blashki et al., 2011; Hayes, Blashki, Wiseman, Burke & Reifels, 2018; Verrinder & Talbot, 2015). The very old and very young; people living with psychosocial disability or chronic health conditions; and financially disadvantaged people are all at increased risk (Altman & Jordan, 2018; Mason, 2011; Running, 2015; Sampson et al., 2013). This in turn leads to increased vulnerability for disadvantaged groups already identified, including Aboriginal and Torres Strait Islander peoples. This occurs due to the intersection of their experiences with increased likelihoods of chronic health conditions, financial disadvantage, and housing insecurity as articulated above. Health social workers must recognise that combinations of these characteristics and factors means that many rural and remote communities are increasingly vulnerable.

There is growing recognition that climate change negatively impacts physical health, mental health, and psychosocial wellbeing (Beggs et al., 2019; Blashki et al., 2011). Australia has experienced changing temperatures and rainfall patterns; and increases in the frequency, duration, and severity of extreme weather events. While the destruction associated with extreme weather events is highly visible, it is the emerging chronic changes that will lead to some non-metropolitan locations becoming uninhabitable, increased food and water insecurity, extended geographic viability of vector-borne diseases such as malaria and dengue fever, and further deterioration in air quality through aero-allergens and pollutants (Anderko, Davies-Cole & Strunk, 2014; Beggs et al., 2019; S. Campbell, 2015; Harley et al., 2011).

The health impacts of climate change are wide and varied. Physical morbidities include increased impacts of cardiovascular and respiratory diseases; diabetes; heat exposure; elevated suicide rates; malnutrition; exposure to zoonotic and vector-borne diseases; increased risk of pre-term birth, stillbirth, and sudden infant death; and deaths and injuries from weather events (Hayes et al., 2018; Hughes & McMichael, 2011; Mills, Gage & Khan, 2010; Vaneckova & Bambrick, 2013; Wang, 2014; Zhang et al., 2018). Climate change exacerbates pre-existing mental illness and may contributes to increased diagnosis of depression, anxiety disorders and post-traumatic stress disorder (Hayes et al., 2018). Related community disruption reduces psychosocial coping strategies and poses a significant threat to disadvantaged populations (Cusack, de Crespigny &

Athanasos, 2011; Hayes et al., 2018; Howard, Agllias, Bevis & Blakemore, 2018). Overall, individual and community wellbeing can be negatively influenced by disruptions to everyday community life; food and water insecurity; displacement from country; increased occupational risk (for example from working in the outdoors); increased domestic and family violence; and reduced air quality including increases in air pollution and aero allergens impacting access to nature and outdoor pursuits (Altman & Jordan, 2018; Beggs et al., 2019; Rychetnik, Sainsbury & Stewart, 2019; Williams et al., 2013).

Health impacts of climate change drive increased demand on public health services, in terms of surge demand during disasters and pandemics (including COVID-19) and day-to-day presentations (Blashki et al., 2011). While research is lacking regarding the explicit impacts for social work, it is clear, that health social work needs to respond to increased climate-related risks. In 2019, the AASW declared a climate change emergency, noting obligations for all social workers given our commitment to social justice and human rights (AASW, 2019). The AASW maintains a position of calling for urgent and immediate action from Australian governments and world influencers (AASW, 2019). Health social workers can drive and contribute to sustained calls for health and broader government policies that aim to reduce carbon reduce greenhouse gas emissions, and to prepare non-metropolitan communities to manage extreme weather events.

Social workers also have a role in working with individuals, families, and communities in adapting to and reducing climate vulnerabilities. At the community level, health social workers can work towards developing 'climate change resilience plans' which address the specific needs of individual localities and their populations (Hayes et al., 2018). At a more direct practice level, health social workers need to be considering climate change vulnerabilities with the people they work with. They need to be asking new questions that help people consider their climate risks and protective factors. Does the patient with chronic kidney disease (known to be vulnerable to extreme heat) have the means in their living environment to keep cool? Can the person access health services without putting themselves at risk of heat exposure – through for example a lack of transport in a hot area. Applying a climate aware lens to biopsychosocial assessments and safe discharge planning is required – and this requires putting the environment back into the person: environment and thinking about *people as place.*

Practice Implications

- Regional, rural, and remote communities are far from homogenous or mono-cultural – there is incredible diversity in the context of some shared characteristics and experiences.
- Social determinants of health and wellbeing need to be addressed to respond to structural drivers of health inequalities, social exclusion, and oppression.
- Cultural safety is imperative when working with diverse groups of individuals and communities – inclusive of Aboriginal and Torres Strait Islander peoples.
- Triple bottom line – understanding the intersection of social, economic, and environmental issues and policies.
- Helpful theoretical lenses include people as place (ecological approaches); intersectionality; and cultural safety.
- Community-embedded practice is imperative – doing with people and communities as opposed to doing to.

Conclusions

Regional, rural, and remote health social work provides opportunities for holistic thinking and generalist and generic practice that are rarely available in major cities. This, along with the diversity of these communities and places, provides a myriad of opportunities for exciting and rewarding social work practice. Adopting *people as place* as the foundational metaphor for social work practice sets the tone for holistic thinking and service delivery. It encourages health social workers to engage with the people and communities served to enable *living well in place*. As a metaphor it helps avoid the unhelpful homogenisation of rural and remote communities and the deficit lens and subsequent narratives that dominate understandings of regional, rural, and remote health. It reminds social workers that the health of different peoples is intrinsically linked to the health of place.

By drawing on Bourke et al.'s (2012) framework for rural and remote health, social workers connect the micro, meso, and macro forces at play in the construction of health in non-metropolitan locations. They are provided with a space in which, as health professionals in the rural locale, they can have agency in contributing to positive, localised responses that go onto further shape and contribute to health in that place. Community-embedded practice, which works with the community strengthening key natural support networks and responding to the unique needs of a particular people and place (Cheers et al., 2007) is essential to this space. Health social workers must embrace cultural safety and recognise the roles they can play in redressing the intersection of racism and multiple oppressions in rural and remote locations.

A confronting obligation for all social workers is climate change. With its links to environmental justice, health social work practice in non-metropolitan spaces must be committed to working with local people and communities in search of sustainable and socially just environments.

Acknowledgement

The authors would like to acknowledge the contribution of social work student, Rebecca Hamlet, for her work regarding the intersections between climate change, health, and health social work.

Key Website Resources

Indigenous Allied Health Alliance (https://iaha.com.au).

National Rural Health Alliance (www.ruralhealth.org.au).

Services for Australian Rural and Remote Allied Health (https://sarrah.org.au).

Social Workers for Climate Action (www.socialworkersforclimateaction.org).

References

AASW. (2019). AASW's policy position on climate change. Retrieved from www.aasw.asn.au/social-policy-advocacy/policy-positions/aasws-policy-position-on-climate-change.

AASW. (2020). Telehealth guide for social workers. Retrieved from www.aasw.asn.au/document/item/12912.

ABS. (2018). *Estimates of Aboriginal and Torres Strait Islander Australians*. ABS.

AIHW. (2019). *Rural and Remote Health Web Report*. AIHW.

Alston, M. (2015). Rural social work. In J. D. Wright (ed.), *International Encyclopedia of the Social & Behavioural Sciences* (2nd ed., Vol. 20, pp. 807–813). Elsevier.

Altman, J. & Jordan, K. (2018). Impact of climate change on indigenous Australians: submission to the Garnaut Climate Change Review. Retrieved from https://openresearch-repository.anu.edu.au/bitstream/1885/148962/1/Altman_Jordan_Garnaut_Review_0.pdf.

Anderko, L., Davies-Cole, J. & Strunk, A. (2014). Identifying populations at risk: interdisciplinary environmental climate change tracking. *Public Health Nursing*, 31(6), 484–491.

Australian Bureau of Statistics. (2018). Australian Statistical Geography Standard (ASGS): volume 5 – remoteness structure. Retrieved from www.abs.gov.au/AUSSTATS/abs@.nsf/Latestproducts/1270.0.55.005Main%20Features15July%202016

Australian Institute of Health and Welfare. (2018). *Australia's Health 2018*. Canberra: AIHW.

Beggs, P. J., Zhang, Y., Bambrick, H., Berry, H. L., Linnenluecke, M. K., Trueck, S., ... Capon, A. G. (2019). The 2019 report of the MJA–Lancet countdown on health and climate change: a turbulent year with mixed progress. *Medical Journal of Australia*, 211(11), 490–491.

Blashki, G., Armstrong, G., Berry, H. L., Weaver, H. J., Hanna, E. G., Bi, P., ... Spickett, J. T. (2011). Preparing health services for climate change in Australia. *Asia Pacific Journal of Public Health*, 23(2_suppl), 133S–143S.

Boetto, H. (2019). Advancing transformative eco-social change: shifting from modernist to holistic foundations. *Australian Social Work*, 72(2), 139–151.

Bohanna, I., Harriss, L., McDonald, M., Cullen, J., Strivens, E., Bird, K., ... Barker, R. (2021). A systematic review of disability, rehabilitation and lifestyle services in rural and remote Australia through the lens of the people-centred health care. *Disability and Rehabilitation*, online ahead of print.

Bourke, L., Humphreys, J. S., Wakerman, J. & Taylor, J. (2012). Understanding rural and remote health: a framework for analysis in Australia. *Health & Place*, 18(3), 496–503.

Bradford, N., Caffery, L. & Smith, A. (2016). Telehealth services in rural and remote Australia: a systematic review of models of care and factors influencing success and sustainability. *Rural and Remote Health*, 16(3808).

Campbell, N., McAllister, L. & Eley, D. (2012). The influence of motivation in recruitment and retention of rural and remote allied health professionals: a literature review. *Rural and Remote Health*, 12(1900).

Campbell, S. (2015). Let's not forget climate change in the food insecurity conversation: why the homeless are most vulnerable. *Health Promotion Journal of Australia*, 26(2), 161.

Cheers, B., Darracott, R. & Lonne, B. (2007). *Social Care Practice in Rural Communities*. Sydney: Federation Press.

Commonwealth of Australia. (2020). *Education in Remote and Complex Environments*. Canberra: Commonwealth of Australia. Retrieved from www.aph.gov.au/Parliamentary_Business/Committees/House/Employment_Education_and_Training/RemoteEducation/Report.

Cox, L., Taua, C., Drummond, A. & Kidd, J. (2020). Enabling cultural safety. In J. Crisp, C. Douglas, G. Rebeiro, D. Waters & E. Plowman (eds), *Potter and Perry's Fundamentals of Nursing* (6th ed., pp. 49–83). Chatswood: Elsevier.

Cusack, L., de Crespigny, C. & Athanasos, P. (2011). Heatwaves and their impact on people with alcohol, drug and mental health conditions: a discussion paper on clinical practice considerations. *Journal of Advanced Nursing*, 67(4), 915–922.

Darracott, R. & Lonne, B. (2017). Rural and remote practice. In K. Ellem, W. H. Chui & J. Wilson (eds), *Social Work and Human Services Best Practice* (2nd ed.). Sydney: Federation Press.

Dominelli, L. (2012). *Green Social Work: From Environmental Crises to Environmental Justice*. Oxford: Polity Press.

Dominelli, L. (2013). Environmental justice at the heart of social work practice: greening the profession. *International Journal of Social Welfare*, 22(4), 431–439.

Duthie, D. (2019). Embedding Indigenous knowledges and cultural safety in social work curricula. *Australian Social Work*, 72(1), 113–116.

Fleming, T., Creedy, D. K. & West, R. (2020). The influence of yarning circles: a cultural safety professional development program for midwives. *Women and Birth*, 33, 175–185.

Fors, M. (2018). Geographical narcissism in psychotherapy: countermapping urban assumptions about power, space, and time. *Psychoanalytic Psychology*, 35(4), 446–453.

Harley, D., Bi, P., Hall, G., Swaminathan, A., Tong, S. & Williams, C. (2011). Climate change and infectious diseases in Australia: future prospects, adaptation options, and research priorities. *Asia Pacific Journal of Public Health*, 23(2_suppl), 54S–66S.

Harvey, E. & Jones, M. (2021). Using complex adaptive systems theory to understand the complexities of hospital social work practice in rural and remote South Australia. *The British Journal of Social Work*, bcab197.

Hayes, K., Blashki, G., Wiseman, J., Burke, S. & Reifels, L. (2018). Climate change and mental health: risks, impacts and priority actions. *International Journal of Mental Health Systems*, 12(1), 28.

Heslop, C., Burns, S. & Lobo, R. (2018). Managing qualitative research as insider-research in small rural communities. *Rural and Remote Health*, 18, 4576.

Howard, A., Agllias, K., Bevis, M. & Blakemore, T. (2018). How social isolation affects disaster preparedness and response in Australia: implications for social work. *Australian Social Work*, 71(4), 392–404.

Hughes, L. & McMichael, T. (producer). (2011). The critical decade: climate change and health. Retrieved from http://climatecommission.gov.au/wp-content/uploads/111129_FINAL-FOR-WEB.pdf.

Hussain, R., Wark, S. & Ryan, P. (2018). Caregiving, employment and social isolation: challenges for rural carers in Australia. *International Journal of Environmental Research and Public Health*, 15, 2267.

Malatzky, C. & Bourke, L. (2016). Re-producing rural health: challenging dominant discourses and the manifestation of power. *Journal of Rural Studies*, 45, 157–164.

Malatzky, C. & Bourke, L. (2018). Different perspectives on the key challenges facing rural health: the challenges of power and knowledge. *Australian Journal of Rural Health*, 26(6), 436–440.

Mason, R. (2011). Confronting uncertainty: lessons from rural social work. *Australian Social Work*, 64(3), 377–394.

Mills, J. N., Gage, K. L. & Khan, A. S. (2010). Potential influence of climate change on vector-borne and zoonotic diseases: a review and proposed research plan. *Environmental Health Perspectives*, 118(11), 1507–1514.

National Rural Health Alliance. (2014). Income inequality experienced by the people of rural and remote Australia: submission to the Senate Inquiry into the Extent of Income Inequality in Australia. Retrieved from www.ruralhealth.org.au/sites/default/files/documents/nrha-policy-document/submissions/sub-income-inequality-inquiry-15-oct-2014.pdf.

OECD. (2016). *Health Workforce Policies in OECD Countries: Right Jobs, Right Skills, Right Places*. Paris: OECD Publishing.

Pease, B. (2013). A history of critical and radical social work. In M. Gray & S. Webb (eds.), *The New Politics of Social Work* (pp. 21–43). Hampshire: Palgrave Macmillan.

Prout, S. (2008). *The Entangled Relationship between Indigenous Spatiality and Government Service Delivery*. CAEPR working paper no. 41/2008. Canberra: Centre for Aboriginal Economic Policy Research, Australian National University.

Rambaree, K. (2020). Environmental social work: implications for accelerating the implementation of sustainable development in social work curricula. *International Journal of Sustainability in Higher Education*, 21(3), 557–574.

Robards, F., Kang, M., Luscombe, G., Hawke, C., Sanci, L., Steinbeck, K., … Usherwood, T. (2020). Intersectionality: social marginalisation and self-reported health status in young people. *International Journal of Environmental Research and Public Health*, 17(21), 8104.

Roberts, P. & Green, B. (2013). Researching rural places: on social justice and rural education. *Qualitative Inquiry*, 19(10), 765–774.

Roberts, P. & Guenther, J. (2021). Framing rural and remote: key issues, debates, definitions, and positions in constructing rural and remote disadvantage. In P. Roberts & M. Fuqua (eds), *Ruraling Education Research* (pp. 13–27). Singapore: Springer.

Running, K. (2015). Towards climate justice: how do the most vulnerable weigh environment–economy trade-offs?. *Social Science Research*, 50, 217–228.

Rural Health Standing Committee. (2011). *National Strategic Framework for Rural and Remote Health*. Canberra: Australian Government. Retrieved from www1.health.gov.au/internet/main/publishing.nsf/Content/national-strategic-framework-rural-remote-health.

Russell, D. & Humphreys, J. (2016). Meeting the primary healthcare needs of small rural communities: lessons for health service planners. *Rural and Remote Health*, 16(3695).

Rychetnik, L., Sainsbury, P. & Stewart, G. (2019). How local health districts can prepare for the effects of climate change: an adaptation model applied to metropolitan Sydney. *Australian Health Review*, 43(6), 601–610.

Sampson, N. R., Gronlund, C. J., Buxton, M. A., Catalano, L., White-Newsome, J. L., Conlon, K. C., … Parker, E. A. (2013). Staying cool in a changing climate: reaching vulnerable populations during heat events. *Global Environmental Change*, 23(2), 475–484.

Tujague, N. A. & Ryan, K. L. (2021). Ticking the box of 'cultural safety' is not enough: why trauma-informed practice is critical to Indigenous healing. *Rural and Remote Health*, 21, 6411.

Vaneckova, P. & Bambrick, H. (2013). Cause-specific hospital admissions on hot days in Sydney, Australia. *PLoS ONE*, 8(2).

Verrinder, G. & Talbot, L. (2015). Rural communities experiencing climate change: a systems approach adaptation. In R. Walker & W. Mason (eds), *Climate Change Adaption for Health and Social Services* (pp. 179–199). Clayton South: CSIRO Publishing.

Wakerman, J., Humphreys, J., Russell, D., Guthridge, S., Bourke, L., Dunbar, T., … Jones, M. P. (2019). Remote health workforce turnover and retention: what are the policy and practice priorities? *Human Resources for Health*, 77(99).

Wakerman, J., Humphreys, J., S, Wells, R., Kuipers, P., Entwistle, P. & Jones, J. (2008). Primary health care delivery models in rural and remote Australia – a systematic review. *BMC Health Services Research*, 8(276).

Wakerman, J. & Humphreys, J. S. (2011). Sustainable primary health care services in rural and remote areas: innovation and evidence. *Australian Journal of Rural Health*, 19(3), 118–124.

Wang, J. (2014). Assessment of the effects of maternal exposure to heatwave on birth outcomes in Brisbane, Australia. PhD, Queensland University of Technology, Brisbane. Retrieved from https://eprints.qut.edu.au/76289/1/Jiajia_Wang_Thesis.pdf.

Wendt, S. (2009). Constructions of local culture and impacts on domestic violence in an Australian rural community. *Journal of Rural Studies*, 25(2), 175–184.

Whelan, J., Millar, L., Bell, C., Russell, C., Grainger, F., Allender, S. & Love, P. (2018). You can't find health food in the bush: poor accessibility, availability and adequacy of food in rural Australia. *International Journal of Environmental Research and Public Health*, 15(10), 2316.

Williams, S., Bi, P., Newbury, J., Robinson, G., Pisaniello, D., Saniotis, A. & Hansen, A. (2013). Extreme heat and health: perspectives from health service providers in rural and remote communities in South Australia. *International Journal of Environmental Research and Public Health*, 10(11).

Zapf, M. K. (2009). *Social Work and the Environment: Understanding People and Place*. Toronto: Canadian Scholars' Press.

Zhang, Y., Beggs, P. J., Bambrick, H., Berry, H. L., Linnenluecke, M. K., Trueck, S., … Capon, A. G. (2018). The MJA–Lancet Countdown on health and climate change: Australian policy inaction threatens lives. *Medical Journal of Australia*, 209(11), 474.

Index

Entries in **bold** refer to tables; entries in *italics* refer to figures.

For Product Safety Concerns and Information please contact our EU representative GPSR@taylorandfrancis.com
Taylor & Francis Verlag GmbH, Kaufingerstraße 24, 80331 München, Germany

www.ingramcontent.com/pod-product-compliance
Lightning Source LLC
LaVergne TN
LVHW060623300926
849162LV00008B/1697